APPLIED NEUROPSYCHOLOGY

Editor-in-Chief
B. P. Uzzell, *Houston, Texas, USA*

Book & Test Review Editor
Nick A. DeFilippis, *Atlanta, Georgia, USA*

Editorial Board

Alfredo Ardila
Miami, Florida, USA

Russell M. Bauer
Gainesville, Florida, USA

Joan C. Borod
New York, New York, USA

Lucia Willadino Braga
Brasilia, Brazil

A. Castro-Caldas
Lisboa, Portugal

John D. Corrigan
Columbus, Ohio, USA

Michael D. Franzen
Pittsburgh, PA, USA

W. Drew Gouvier
Baton Rouge, Louisiana, USA

Peter W. Halligan
Cardiff, UK

H. Julia Hannay
Houston, Texas, USA

Mary Ellen Hayden
Dallas, Texas, USA

Merrill C. Hiscock
Houston, Texas, USA

Muriel D. Lezak
Portland, Oregon, USA

Lisa A. Morrow
Pittsburgh, Pennsylvania, USA

Feggy Ostrosky-Solis
Mexico City, Mexico

Cecil R. Reynolds
College Station, Texas, USA

Jarl A. Risberg
Lund, Sweden

Ronald M. Ruff
San Francisco, California, USA

Mark Sherer
Jackson, Mississippi, USA

E. Arthur Shores
Sydney, Australia

Tom M. Tombaugh
Ottawa, Ontario, Canada

Michael G. Tramontana
Nashville, Tennessee, USA

Rodney D. Vanderploeg
Tampa, Florida, USA

Nils R. Varney
Iowa City, Iowa, USA

Juhani Vilkki
Helsinki, Finland

J. T. Lindsay Wilson
Stirling, Scotland, UK

Journal Production Editor
Rick Maffei
Lawrence Erlbaum Associates, Inc.

Aim and Scope: *Applied Neuropsychology* publishes clinical neuropsychological articles concerning assessment, brain functioning and neuroimaging, neuropsychological treatment, and rehabilitation. Full-length articles and brief communications are included. Case studies and reviews, carefully assessing the nature, course, or treatment of clinical neuropsychological dysfunctions in the context of the scientific literature, are suitable. Preference is given to papers of clinical relevance to others in the field. Clarity and soundness of reporting will ensure rapid publication.

Applied Neuropsychology is abstracted or indexed in *Index Medicus/MEDLINE; PsycINFO/Psychological Abstracts; EMBASE/Excerpta Medica; Cambridge Scientific Abstracts: Health & Safety Science; EBSCOhost Products; Risk Abstracts; Linguistics and Language Behavior Abstracts; ScienceDirect Navigator.* Microform copies of this journal are available through Bell & Howell Information and Learning, P.O. Box 1346, Ann Arbor, MI 48106–1346 USA. For more information, call 1-800-521-0600, x2888.

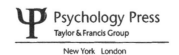

Ψ Psychology Press
Taylor & Francis Group

New York   London

Applied Neuropsychology
2004, Vol. 11, No. 1, 1–3

INTRODUCTION

Cultural Diversity and Neuropsychology: An Uneasy Relationship in a Time of Change

Ruben J. Echemendia

Psychological and Neurobehavioral Associates, State College, Pennsylvania, USA

The United States is rapidly becoming a multicultural society. It is hard to overlook this fact as you walk in our cities, read newspapers and magazines, watch television, and examine what is being taught in our schools. The demographic data are quite clear. The U.S. Census (U.S. Bureau of the Census, 2000) indicates that, for those people who identified themselves as belonging to one race, the United States is 75.1% White, 12.5% Hispanic or Latino, 12.3% Black or African American, 3.6% Asian or Asian American, 0.9% American Indian or Alaska Native, 0.1% Native Hawaiian or Pacific Islander, and 5.5% "other." Approximately 2.4% of the population identified themselves as belonging to two or more races.

The White population is growing at a far slower rate than other ethnic or racial groups. For example, between the years 1990 and 2000, the White (non-Hispanic) population grew at a rate of 8.6%, the Black population grew at 21.5%, Hispanics/Latinos increased their numbers by 57.9%, American Indians/Alaska Natives increased by 110.3%, the Asian population grew by 72.2%, Native Hawaiians increased by 139.5%, and "others" increased by 88.9%. More important, by the year 2050, it is projected that 13.3% of the U.S. population will be foreign born. Non-Hispanic Whites will make up 52.8% of the population, Hispanics will account for 24.5% of the population, Blacks or African Americans will represent 14.7% of the population, American Indians will account for 1.1% of the population, and Asians/Pacific Islanders will account for 9.3% of the population (U.S. Bureau of the Census, 2000).

These population data and projections point to significant variability within the U.S. population. There is also a great deal of variability within each of the cultural groups. Harris, Echemendia, Ardila, and Rosselli (2001) pointed out that there are 556 federally recognized American Indian tribes and Alaska Native entities and that 135 American Indian and 20 Alaska Native languages have been documented. Hispanics in the United States share a common language, but trace their origins to a wide range of countries such as Mexico, Puerto Rico, Cuba, the Dominican Republic, Argentina, Columbia, Spain, Honduras, Panama, and many others. In fact, the United States now has the fifth-largest Spanish-speaking population in the world (Ardila, Rodriguez-Menendez, & Rosselli, 2002). Wong and Fujii point out that the U.S. Bureau of the Census divides Asian Americans into six discrete groups (Asian Indian, Chinese, Filipino, Japanese, Korean, and Vietnamese). However, there are 32 uniquely identifiable cultural groups within these larger groups.

Racial classification is even more complex. Although the U.S. Bureau of the Census generally recognizes three distinct races (Black, White, Mongolian), interracial unions, either forced, as in times of colonization, or by consent, have led to a largely multiracial society. In this context, Manly, Byrd, Tourajdi, and Stern view racial classifications as "social/political classifications as opposed to scientifically or genetically defined categories."

The diversity among people in the United States as described here is further complicated by the addition of many demographic variables that cut across each of these ethnic/cultural groupings. These variables include acculturation, number of years in the United States, education (current and country of origin), quality of education, socioeconomic standing (current and

Requests for reprints should be sent to Ruben J. Echemendia, 119 South Burrowes Street, Suite 707, State College, PA 16801, USA. E-mail: rechemendia@adelphia.net

country of origin), reason for immigration, and English-language fluency, to name but a few.

In contrast to the cultural diversity observed in the U.S. population, neuropsychologists in the United States are almost exclusively White and English-speaking and use largely Eurocentric models of mind–body relationships. The lack of cultural congruence between the population served by neuropsychologists and the neuropsychologists themselves is not specific to neuropsychology; the same pattern is observed in psychology as a whole. It is interesting to note that the same pattern has not been observed among our medical colleagues (see Hill-Briggs, Evans, & Norman).

The goal of this special issue is to examine salient aspects of culture and neuropsychology and to assist in bringing the issue of culture and cultural diversity to the forefront of neuropsychological discussions. Because of space limitations, this special issue only "scratches the surface" of the many issues that must be addressed by our field. Indeed, we likely raise many more questions than we are able to answer. Raising these questions allows others to further the discourse and to begin the many empirical investigations necessary for us, as a profession, to adequately serve the needs of the population that entrusts its care to us.

The title of this issue suggests that an uneasy relationship exists between neuropsychology and culture. Part of the tension in this relationship may reflect the fact that neuropsychology is a relatively new discipline. As with any new discipline, the initial emphasis is on "bedrock" issues such as developing a professional identity, developing tests, identifying brain–behavior relationships, and the like. Through the process of maturation, the field has developed to a point where there is ample room for including cultural variables as one of our core sets of variables. Growing interest in cultural variables is apparent in the increased number of journal articles that examine culture, increased opportunities for training through workshops at meetings such as the National Academy of Neuropsychology, appointment of standing committees on issues of diversity in all three of the major neuropsychological associations (National Academy of Neuropsychology, American Psychological Association [APA]–Division 40, International Neuropsychological Society), and increased visibility of cultural issues at national meetings. For example, the most recent APA convention (Toronto, 2003) featured a Division 40 program that was significant for the number, quality, and variety of cultural entries. Unfortunately, the growth in scientific and clinical interest in cultural variables has not translated into increased numbers of U.S. ethnic neuropsychologists.

The selection of articles for this issue was geared toward providing a broad sample of theoretical, empirical, and applied perspectives across a broad representation of ethnic/racial groups. I chose to invite authors who span the range of professional development: established senior neuropsychologists as well as mid-career and junior-level colleagues.

Hill-Briggs et al. begin by describing the demographic characteristics of U.S. neuropsychologists. In the process of collecting their data, an interesting and poignant issue became apparent: Neuropsychological organizations do not routinely gather ethnic/racial data on their members. This finding, by itself, raises many interesting questions and important challenges. Is the fact that these data are not routinely gathered simply a reflection of the marginalization that ethic minorities experience within neuropsychology? Is it benign neglect? Does it reflect fear among these organizations that asking these questions may lead to legal challenges? Might it suggest that tackling issues related to cultural diversity is too complex and hence should be avoided? Or is it some combination of all of these?

In this issue, Echemendia and Harris present additional data from a national survey of neurologists first published in 1997 (Ardila et al., 2002; Echemendia, Harris, Congett, Diaz, & Puente, 1997). These new data reveal that U.S. neuropsychologists conduct neuropsychological assessments on monolingual and bilingual Spanish-speaking patients in much the same way they conduct evaluations on English-speaking patients. Generally, the same tests and norms are used. Sometimes, the neuropsychologists or their translators translate the tests, and, oftentimes, clinical judgment is exercised in place of clearly inappropriate norms when interpreting test data. These data highlight the need for Spanish language neuropsychological tests with appropriately derived normative data.

Wong and Fuji describe the diversity of Asian peoples and help us understand their cultural experiences within the United States. This article not only describes the heterogeneity of Asian cultures, but also helps the reader by providing practical suggestions with regard to the selection and administration of neuropsychological instruments with this population.

Brown, McCauley, Levin, Contant, and Boake examined ethnic differences in the recovery process after traumatic brain injury and identified factors relevant to enhancing recovery among Whites, African Americans, and Hispanics/Latino Americans. Their data provide interesting insights into differences in health perception and the importance of using cultural variables in the assessment of recovery after head injury.

Llorente, Turcich, and Lawrence undertook an interesting study that examined the neuropsychological performance of White and African American HIV-1 positive children. The differences observed among these children provide fertile ground for discussions regarding the interactions of disease processes, genetics, and demographic variables.

Manly et al. provide a new perspective on ethnic differences in neuropsychological test performance. They begin by providing an informative discussion on the historical views of racial differences in cognitive tests and challenge the use of ethnic-specific norms, arguing that the "use of separate norms leaves ethnic differences in test performance unexplained, unexamined, and thus not understood." Dr. Manly and her team of researchers have published a series of articles based on systematic research with elder African American populations. In the article in this issue, Manly and her colleagues show that acculturation and education play a critical role in the neuropsychological performance of elderly African Americans. This article underscores the need to examine education and acculturation for all patients, even those for whom acculturation is assumed because they have been long-time residents of the United States and for whom English is their native language.

Taken together, the articles in this special issue help further our understanding that ethnic and cultural variables are important not only in research design, but also in clinical practice. These articles urge clinicians to make cultural variables an integral component of any neuropsychological assessment and to examine clinical data in the context of the patient's ethnic and cultural background. A challenge to all clinical neuropsychologists is to include a section in *every* neuropsychological report entitled "Demographic/Cultural Background." This section would be just as appropriate for the White, Jewish New York banker as it would be for the rural Pennsylvania farmer or the recent Mexican immigrant. All of us, patients and neuropsychologists alike, have cultural backgrounds. The ecological validity of our interpretations will be enhanced if neuropsychologists become aware of and appreciate the effect of these cultural variables. At the very least, it would allow our patients to feel that we understand them better. Although cultural variables have been assigned largely to "error variance" in the past, neuropsychology can take significant strides forward by identifying the proportion of this variance that can be captured by cultural variables.

In closing, I thank Dr. Barbara Uzzell for the opportunity to serve as the guest editor for this special issue and for maintaining her dedication to issues of culture in neuropsychology. I also thank all of the authors who contributed their hard work and effort to this issue.

References

Ardila, A., Rodriguez-Menendez, G., & Rosselli, M. (2002). Current issues in neuropsychological assessment with Hispanics/Latinos. In R. Ferraro (Ed.), *Minority and cross-cultural aspects of neuropsychological assessment* (pp. 161–179). Lisse, The Netherlands: Swets & Zeitlinger. Echemendia, R. J., Harris, J. G., Congett, S. M., Diaz, L. M., & Puente, A. (1997). Neuropsychological training and practices with Hispanics: A national survey. *Clinical Neuropsychologist, 11*, 229–243.

Harris, J., Echemendia, R. J., Ardila, A., & Rosselli, M. (2001). Cross-cultural cognitive and neuropsychological assessment. In H. J. J. Andrews & D. Saklofske (Eds.), *Handbook of psychoeducational assessment* (pp. 392–414). San Diego, CA: Academic.

U. S. Bureau of the Census (2000). Population estimates. Retrieved January 10, 2004 from http://www.census.gov

Applied Neuropsychology
2004, Vol. 11, No. 1, 4–12

ARTICLES

Neuropsychological Test Use With Hispanic/Latino[1] Populations in the United States: Part II of a National Survey

Ruben J. Echemendia

Psychological and Neurobehavioral Associates, State College, Pennsylvania

Josette G. Harris

Departments of Psychiatry and Neurology
University of Colorado School of Medicine

A national survey was conducted with the aim of characterizing the status of neuropsychological practice with Hispanic[1] individuals in the United States. In an earlier article (Echemendia, Harris, Congett, Diaz, & Puente, 1997), survey findings were presented concerning the characteristics of neuropsychologists who work with Hispanic populations, specific graduate and postgraduate preparation to provide services to culturally diverse groups, and predictors of self-rated competence to work with Hispanic people. In this article, additional results from the survey are presented. Specifically, these results concern reported use of standardized and nonstandardized measures to assess Hispanic people, with particular emphasis on assessment practices with monolingual versus bilingual patients and the use of norms for clinical interpretation.

To present these findings in the proper context, it is important first to address briefly some of the pertinent issues with regard to neuropsychological assessment of culturally or linguistically diverse people. Although the need to consider and address cultural variables is clearly outlined in ethical standards and practice guidelines (American Psychological Association [APA], 1990, 2002), various issues may interfere with the clinician's full consideration of such variables in the assessment of neurobehavioral functions. For example, neur-

opsychologists may be poorly informed regarding the extent to which cultural factors are relevant or may exert an influence on neuropsychological test scores. This may be as much a function of relatively limited published research in the area of cultural neuropsychology as it is the application of untested assumptions of "general" neurobehavioral principles to culturally and linguistically diverse people. Although some of these assumptions may yet prove to be valid, many remain untested. Specific aspects of culture, such as experience living in the United States, country of education, and preferred language, are increasingly being identified as potent variables that affect neuropsychological performance (Harris, Tulsky, & Schultheis, 2003).

With regard to language, little systematic attention has been given to the assessment of language proficiency or competence and the implications for neuropsychological assessment. Standard measures that have been available for some time are not widely used among neuropsychologists and are better known among psychoeducational providers for use in the identification of school-age English Language Learners and Limited English Proficiency students (Language Assessment Scale, 1990, 1994; Stanford English Language Proficiency Test, 1990; Woodcock-Muñoz Language Survey, Woodcock & Muñoz-Sandoval, 1993; Idea Proficiency Test). The focus of these measures tends to be on the measurement of comprehension, vocabulary, syntax, and other fundamental language skills important to educational testing and educational services planning and intervention. Neuropsychologists may base their decisions regarding the appropriateness

---

[1]To simplify presentation, the terms *Hispanic* and *Latino* are used interchangeably throughout this article. *Latino* is also used to refer to both Latinos and Latinas.

Requests for reprints should be sent to Ruben J. Echemendia, 119 South Burrowes Street, Suite 707, State College, PA 16801, USA. E-mail: rechemendia@adelphia.net

of using English language verbal measures on the examinee's ability to participate in casual conversation with the examiner, but examinees may at times overstate their mastery of English in an effort to gain acceptance by peers and others in the community, including professionals with whom they interact. Examiners may rely on an arbitrary standard for administering a test in English, such as the length of time an individual has resided in the United States. The latter variable, in particular, may correlate with language proficiency, but second language learning is very complex, and a multitude of factors influence patterns of use, proficiency, and perceived competence (Ardila, 1998; Harris, Echemendia, Ardila, & Rosselli, 2001).

Finally, these survey results must be presented in the context of the current state of affairs regarding the underrepresentation of culturally diverse providers in all specialties of psychology. Perhaps clinicians approach the assessment of culturally diverse people with the realization that their resources, knowledge base, and experiences are limited, but nevertheless, they feel compelled, because of a lack of available providers (e.g., Hispanic, Spanish-speaking neuropsychologists) and pressure from referral sources, to meet the needs of these people. With the continued growth of the linguistic and cultural diversity of the U.S. population, such demands, which outstrip resources, are likely to continue to rise. Thus, it becomes imperative to identify the current practices in the provision of neuropsychological services to various subgroups and people living within the larger U.S. population, to understand the strengths and weaknesses of those approaches, and to ultimately develop more effective tools and methodologies for meeting the challenges that our societal diversity presents.

Method

The methods used in this study have been described in detail elsewhere (Echemendia et al., 1997). A comprehensive survey concerning professional training and clinical practices with Hispanic, Spanish-speaking patients was mailed to a national sample of neuropsychologists. A total of 911 surveys were returned. The sample was deemed to be representative of U.S. neuropsychologists on the basis of a variety of demographic and practice factors (Echemendia et al., 1997). The survey was divided into two components. The first component addressed the cultural background and training of neuropsychologists; their ability to speak, read, and write in Spanish; their experiences working with Lat-

inos, Spanish-speaking populations; and their self-perceived competence to work with these populations. The second portion of the survey, which is the focus of this article, examined the instruments and norms used by U.S. neuropsychologists when working with Spanish-speaking populations. Only those neuropsychologists who reported experience working with Hispanics completed this portion of the survey.

Respondents were asked to report the tests they use and then to indicate whether they use each test with monolinguals (Spanish only) or bilinguals. They also were asked to indicate the version of the test that they use: (a) published English language test, (b) nonpublished personal verbatim translation of an English test, (c) nonpublished Spanish culturally adapted translation (not a verbatim translation) of a published English test, or (d) published Spanish language test. The respondents were asked to indicate whether they use published norms from an English-speaking sample, published norms from a Spanish-speaking sample, or clinical judgment to interpret the test results. A list of the most commonly used tests in neuropsychology was provided, with columns for these variables as well as space for respondents to include any test used that was not listed.

Results

A total of 475 (52%) neuropsychologists completed the second portion of the survey. Table 1 presents the 10 most frequently reported tests used with bilingual and monolingual Hispanics. As can be seen, the Wechsler Adult Intelligence Scale (WAIS) is the most widely used test within each group. Please note that the "combined" category is not a simple addition of the monolingual and bilingual categories. This category indicates that the neuropsychologist used the test with both monolingual and bilingual groups. Some neuropsychologists use tests with only monolinguals, others with only bilinguals, and some use the combination. Similarly, some neuropsychologists may practice with only bilinguals, whereas others may practice exclusively with monolinguals.

Table 1 reveals remarkable consistency among the tests used with the different language groups. The WAIS, Trail Making Test (Trails), Wechsler Memory Scale, Wisconsin Card Sorting Test (WCST), Rey Complex Figure Test, California Verbal Learning Test (CVLT), and Boston Naming Test (BNT) were common to all three groups. The combined group also made use of the Ravens Progressive Matrices and the Symbol

Table 1. *Comparison of Tests With the Highest Frequency of Endorsement Across Groups*

Test Name (Frequency)		
Combined[a]	**Monolingual**	**Bilingual**
WAIS (461)	WAIS (110)	WAIS (283)
Trails (366)	Trails (57)	WMS (195)
WMS (302)	WMS (55)	Trails (180)
WCST (269)	CVLT (46)	CVLT (171)
RCFT (258)	S/P (43)	WCST (149)
CVLT (253)	MMSE (41)	Log. Mem (141)
S/P (228)	Log. Mem (38)	BNT (135)
BNT (215)	WCST (38)	HRB (126)
Ravens (212)	BNT (35)	RCFT (120)
SDMT (159)	RCFT (35)	Stroop (119)

Note: WAIS = Wechsler Adult Intelligence Scale; Trails = Trail Making Test; WMS = Wechsler Memory Scale; WCST = Wisconsin Card Sorting Test; CVLT = California Verbal Learning Test; RCFT = Rey Complex Figure Test; S/P = Reitan-Klove Sensory Perceptual Exam; MMSE = Mini Mental Status Examination; Log. Mem = Logical Memory (WMS); BNT = Boston Naming Test, HRB = Halstead-Reitan Battery; Ravens = Ravens Progressive Matrices; SDMT = Symbol Digit Modalities Test.
[a]The combined group is not a total of the monolingual and bilingual groups.

Table 2. *Neuropsychological Test Usage in the General Population—Tests With the Highest Use Endorsement*

Test	Endorsement
WAIS–R	86
Wisconsin Card Sorting	73
Boston Naming Test	63
Rey-Osterrieth Complex Figure	60
Trail Making Test	59
Wechsler Memory Scale	49
Token Test	49
Controlled Oral Word Association	48
Rey Auditory Verbal Learning	46
Finger Tapping	46
Ravens Progressive Matrices	45
Stroop Color–Word Test	45

Note: WAIS–R = Wechsler Adult Intelligence Scale–Revised. From "Neuropsychological Test Usage," by M. Butler, P. Retzlaff, and R. Vanderploeg, 1991, *Professional Psychology: Research and Practice, 22*, p. 511–512. Copyright © 1991 by the American Psychological Association. Adapted with permission.

Digit Modalities Test. Those neuropsychologists working with monolinguals also reported using the Reitan–Klove Sensory Perceptual Exam (S/P) and the Mini Mental Status Examination (MMSE). Neuropsychologists working with bilinguals reported using the Halstead–Reitan Battery (HRB) and the Stroop Color–Word test, among the most frequently used tests.

This pattern of test use with Hispanic, Spanish-speakers is quite consistent with that used in the general population (Butler, Retzlaff, & Vanderploeg, 1991; Table 2). The only tests endorsed more frequently with the general population were the Token Test, the Controlled Oral Word Association Test, and the Finger Tapping Test. The Token Test was the 11th most frequently used test among both monolinguals and bilinguals in our survey.

We examined whether test selection varied as a function of the neuropsychologist's self-perceived level of competence to work with Hispanics. Neuropsychologists were asked to rate their competence to work with Latinos on a 7-point Likert scale ranging from 1 (*not at all competent*) to 4 (*somewhat competent*) to 7 (*extremely competent*). Echemendia et al. (1997) reported that 22% of the sample felt not all competent to work with Hispanics, and 1.4% felt extremely competent. Approximately 82% of the sample fell in the marginally to somewhat competent range (scale points 2 through 4). Table 3 lists the five tests with the highest frequency of use, with monolinguals and bilinguals as a

Table 3. *Neuropsychological Test Use With Monolingual and Bilingual Spanish Speakers by Neuropsychologists' Self-Rate Level of Competence*

Population	Low Competence—< 4	Midpoint—4	High Competence—> 4
Monolinguals	WAIS	WAIS	WAIS
	Trails/Ravens	WCST	WMS
	MMSE	CVLT/Trails/RCFT	Trails/CVLT
	WMS	WMS	S/P
	Bender/DSMT/WCST	Log. Mem/Let Canc/S/P	Log. Mem
Bilinguals	WAIS	WAIS	WAIS
	WMS	CVLT	WMS
	Trails	WCST	Trails
	CVLT	WMS/BNT	CVLT
	WCST	Trails	HRB

Note: More than one test entry on a line indicates a tie in the frequency of endorsement. WAIS = Wechsler Adult Intelligence Scale; Trails = Trail Making Test; Ravens = Ravens Progressive Matrices; WCST = Wisconsin Card Sorting Test; WMS = Wechsler Memory Scale; MMSE = Mini Mental Status Examination; CVLT = California Verbal Learning Test; RCFT = Rey Complex Figure Test; S/P = Reitan-Klove Sensory Perceptual Exam; DSMT = Digit Symbol Modalities Test; Log. Mem = Logical Memory (WMS); Let Canc = Letter/Number Cancellation; BNT = Boston Naming Test; HRB = Halstead-Reitan Battery.

function of the respondent's self-rated competence. For the purposes of this analysis, respondents were grouped into three categories: low competence (less than 4 on the competence scale), moderate competence (4), and high competence (greater than 4). All groups endorsed the WAIS with the highest frequency, regardless of competence level or examinee language (i.e., monolingual or bilingual). Across competence levels, there appears to be consistent endorsement of tests used, although there is variability in the ranking of the tests within each group. The low-competence group endorsed the Bender–Gestalt more than any other group. The group that viewed itself as highly competent reported using the HRB with bilinguals, whereas the other groups did not.

As was the case with competence, there was marked variability in reported Spanish language proficiency in this sample. Some neuropsychologists were bilingual and bicultural; others were unable to speak Spanish at all. neuropsychologists were asked to rate their ability to speak, read, and understand Spanish on a 7-point Likert scale ranging from 1 (*not at all*) to 4 (*adequate*) to 7 (*completely fluent*). We divided the group into high and low Spanish proficiency using a median split of the simple composite of the three language proficiency items. Few differences were identified between the two proficiency groups (Table 4); the exception was that the low-proficiency group endorsed the S/P with monolinguals, and the high-proficiency group used the MMSE and the BNT with monolinguals. The low-proficiency group used the WCST more often with bilinguals, and

the high-proficiency group used the Stroop Color–Word test and the HRB more often with bilinguals.

Given the variability in language proficiency and the fact that each of these neuropsychologists has worked with Spanish-speaking patients, we examined the neuropsychologists' reliance on translators as a function of their own Spanish language proficiency (see Table 5). As would be expected, neuropsychologists reporting low Spanish language proficiency used translators more frequently than neuropsychologists reporting high Spanish proficiency. It is interesting to note that 38% of the low-proficiency group used translators all or some of the time with monolingual Spanish patients, but rarely used translators with bilinguals. In contrast, even the neuropsychologists who were highly proficient in Spanish used translators at times with both monolinguals and bilinguals.

The process of test development and adaptation is an important consideration in cultural neuropsychology. It is essential to ascertain whether the test is a translation of an English language test, whether the test was normed in the target population, and whether the test was conceptualized and developed or adapted with a specific ethnic or cultural group. Table 6 presents the 10 most frequently endorsed tests used with bilinguals and the test versions reported. Respondents were given the choice between the (a) published English language test, (b) nonpublished personal verbatim translation of an English test, (c) nonpublished Spanish culturally adapted translation (not a verbatim translation) of an English test, or (d) published Spanish language version. Overall, the published English version of the test was most frequently used. However, there was considerable variability among the test versions. Although the WAIS was the most frequently endorsed, the published English version was used only 58% of the time. In contrast, the English version of the Logical Memory subtest was used 96% of the time, the English version of the Stroop Color–Word test was used 96% of the time, and the English version of the HRB was used 61% of the time.

Table 4. *Neuropsychological Test Use as a Function of the Neuropsychologist's Proficiency With Spanish*

	Language Proficiency	
Population	Low	High
Monolingual	WAIS	WAIS
	Trails	WMS
	CVLT	Trails
	WMS	MMSE/CVLT
	S/P	BNT
Bilingual	WAIS	WAIS
	WMS	WMS
	Trails	CVLT
	CVLT	Trails
	WCST	Stroop/HRB

Note: More than one test entry on a line indicates a tie in the frequency of endorsement. WAIS = Wechsler Adult Intelligence Scale; Trails = Trail Making Test; WMS = Wechsler Memory Scale; CVLT = California Verbal Learning Test; MMSE = Mini Mental Status Examination; S/P = Reitan-Klove Sensory Perceptual Exam; BNT = Boston Naming Test; WCST = Wisconsin Card Sorting Test; HRB = Halstead-Reitan Battery.

Table 5. *Use of Translators as a Function of Neuropsychologists' Spanish Language Proficiency*

	Language Proficiency	
Population	Low	High
Monolingual	62% Yes	5% Yes
	18% No	88% No
	20% Sometimes	12% Sometimes
Bilingual	5% Yes	0% Yes
	67% No	90% No
	28% Sometimes	10% Sometimes

Table 6. *Neuropsychological Test Version Used With Bilingual Latinos*

Test	Frequency	Percentages Published English Version	Verbatim Translation	Culturally Adapted	Published Spanish Version
WAIS	283	58	20	10	12
WMS	195	59	31	10	< 1
Trails	180	73	21	5	1
CVLT	171	67	21	10	2
WCST	149	74	24	< 1	< 1
Log. Mem	141	96	2	1	1
BNT	141	73	26	< 1	< 1
HRB	126	61	37	< 1	< 1
RCFT	120	61	37	< 1	1
Stroop	111	96	3	0	1

Note: WAIS = Wechsler Adult Intelligence Scale; WMS = Wechsler Memory Scale; Trails = Trail Making Test; CVLT = California Verbal Learning Test; WCST = Wisconsin Card Sorting Test; Log. Mem = Logical Memory (WMS); BNT = Boston Naming Test; HRB = Halstead-Reitan Battery; RCFT = Rey Complex Figure Test.

Table 7. *Neuropsychological Test Version Used With Monolingual Latinos*

Test	Frequency	Percentages Published English Version	Verbatim Translation	Culturally Adapted	Published Spanish Version
WAIS	110	6	29	13	52
Trails	57	14	61	18	7
WMS	55	13	56	24	7
CVLT	46	2	65	26	7
S/P	43	12	63	19	7
MMSE	41	7	68	12	12
Log. Mem	38	0	53	37	11
WCST	38	3	76	21	0
BNT	35	6	46	40	9
RCFT	35	6	77	11	6

Note: WAIS = Wechsler Adult Intelligence Scale; Trails = Trail Making Test; WMS = Wechsler Memory Scale; CVLT = California Verbal Learning Test; S/P = Reitan-Klove Sensory Perceptual Exam; MMSE = Mini Mental Status Examination; Log. Mem = Logical Memory (WMS); WCST = Wisconsin Card Sorting Test; BNT = Boston Naming Test; RCFT = Rey Complex Figure Test.

Direct verbatim translations of tests were used more frequently than culturally adapted translations. Published Spanish language versions of the tests were rarely used.

Table 7 presents the 10 most frequently endorsed tests and the version of the tests used with monolingual Spanish speakers. In contrast to the bilingual data, only 6% of the neuropsychologists used the published English version of the Wechsler scales with monolinguals, 29% used a personally translated version of the test, and 13% used a cultural adaptation. The 6% that endorsed the use of the English test without translation (with people who speak only Spanish) is remarkable. This cannot be explained by assuming that this 6% is administering only the performance subtests because only a few people reported using this subset of tests. Across all tests, it appears that a verbatim translation is more frequently

used than a culturally adapted translation. Approximately 52% of the group endorsed using a published Spanish version of the WAIS. Even though there are concerns with the normative data in at least one Spanish version of the WAIS (e.g., Melendez, 1994), the fact that 52% use a Spanish alternative suggests that neuropsychologists will use Spanish language tests if they are published and available.

It is important to understand which normative samples are used to interpret the results of neuropsychological tests when they are administered to monolingual and bilingual Spanish speakers. Generally, practitioners who work with patients who are non-native English speakers are discouraged from using norms based on native English speakers or are encouraged to interpret results and in some way reflect the patient's level of English proficiency (American Educational Research

Association, 1999). Respondents were asked to identify whether they use "English" language norms (generated with examinees tested in English) or "Spanish" language norms based on Spanish-speaking normative samples or whether they use their clinical judgment instead of using norms. Tables 8 and 9 present these data for the 10 most often endorsed tests for each group. Table 8 reveals consistency in the use of normative data with bilingual speakers. On average, neuropsychologists use "English" norms approximately 67% of the time and clinical judgment 31% of the time when interpreting test data from bilinguals. They use "Spanish" language norms approximately 2% of the time. Table 9

Table 8. *Norms Used to Interpret Neuropsychological Tests With Bilingual Hispanics*

Test (Frequency)	Normative Data (Percentages)		
	English	Spanish	Clinical Judgment
WAIS (264)	68	4	28
WMS (176)	67	5	28
Trails (170)	66	2	32
CVLT (156)	65	2	33
WCST (137)	71	1	28
Log. Mem. (141)	64	1	35
BNT (135)	65	2	33
HRB (121)	69	0	31
RCFT (103)	64	4	32
Stroop (102)	71	1	28

Note: WAIS = Wechsler Adult Intelligence Scale; WMS = Wechsler Memory Scale; Trails = Trail Making Test; CVLT = California Verbal Learning Test; WCST = Wisconsin Card Sorting Test; Log. Mem = Logical Memory (WMS); BNT = Boston Naming Test; HRB = Halstead-Reitan Battery; RCFT = Rey Complex Figure Test.

Table 9. *Norms Used to Interpret Neuropsychological Tests With Monolingual Spanish Speakers*

Test (Frequency)	Normative Data (Percentages)		
	English	Spanish	Clinical Judgment
WAIS (75)	6	64	29
Trails (40)	20	0	80
WMS (16)	18	24	59
CVLT (13)	31	23	46
MMSE (15)	20	25	55
WCST (15)	20	30	50
RCFT (12)	25	25	50
Log. Mem (11)	18	18	64
S/P (10)	40	0	60
BNT (9)	29	0	71

Note: WAIS = Wechsler Adult Intelligence Scale; Trails = Trail Making Test; WMS = Wechsler Memory Scale; CVLT = California Verbal Learning Test; MMSE = Mini Mental Status Examination; WCST = Wisconsin Card Sorting Test; RCFT = Rey Complex Figure Test; Log. Mem = Logical Memory (WMS); S/P = Reitan-Klove Sensory Perceptual Exam; BNT = Boston Naming Test.

presents the interpretive approaches used with monolingual Spanish speakers. These data reveal greater variability. For example, clinical judgment is used 80% of the time when interpreting the Trails, but only 29% of the time when interpreting the Wechsler scales. Similarly, English language norms are used only 6% of the time with the Wechsler scales, but 31% of the time with the CVLT. On average, English norms are used 23% of the time, clinical judgment is used 57% of the time, and Spanish norms are used 20% of the time.

Discussion

Cuellar (1998) held the view that neuropsychology has largely ignored the importance of culture on neuropsychological test performance. Spanish-speaking populations are one of the largest growing ethnic groups in the United States and represent a broad range of peoples who trace their origins to a variety of Spanish countries (Ardila, Rodriguez-Menendez, & Rosselli, 2002; Echemendia & Julian, 2002). This variability in nationality adds complexity to an already difficult situation: How do U.S. neuropsychologists prepare for and deliver services to a Spanish-speaking population expected to number 98,229,000 by the year 2050, a 213% increase from the year 2000 estimates (U.S. Bureau of the Census, 2000).

To capture a snapshot in time of neuropsychological practices with Spanish speakers, neuropsychologists across the United States were surveyed, and data were obtained regarding their professional training and clinical experiences working with Hispanic populations. The results from the first part of this survey have been reported already (Echemendia et al., 1997). The data from the second part of that survey are presented here. The patterns of test use and practices captured by this survey in 1994 are still believed to be applicable today, given a lag in new test releases for Spanish speakers by major test publishers.

The data obtained from this survey indicate that the tests used by U.S. neuropsychologists with bilingual and monolingual Spanish speakers differ little from the tests used with the general population. Indeed, the Wechsler scales were the most widely used tests across all language groups. The consistent use of the WAIS speaks to the popularity of the tests and the confidence and comfort level neuropsychologists have with the tests. It also may speak to the ease of accessibility of the WAIS. The finding that a large percentage of the time, clinicians use the English language version of a test, or a verbatim translation, along with the finding that practitioners often apply the norms developed on English speakers regardless of the examinee's linguistic status, raises the question of whether neuropsychologists largely downplay the effects of culture and language on neuropsychological test performance. Although ethical and professional standards and guidelines (American Educational Research Association, 1999; APA, 1990, 1992, 2002) direct neuropsychologists to carefully consider and evaluate cultural and linguistic variables and to carefully consider test and nontest alternatives, the data presented here suggest that these issues are not given much weight. Alternatively, it may signify that practitioners are desperately "filling in the gaps" because suitable alternative methods and empirical data to guide practice are lacking (Harris et al., 2003).

The data collected from this survey clearly point to wide variability among neuropsychologists in their preparation to work with Spanish-speaking populations. However, when test use was analyzed by level of self-perceived competence, there were few differences among those neuropsychologists who perceived themselves as competent to work with this population and those who did not. Again, this finding may reflect the lack of available tests for use with this population, inaccurate estimations by neuropsychologists of their own competence levels, or the belief that cultural and linguistic factors are not salient issues.

Similar to the variability that existed among neuropsychologists regarding their preparation to work with Latinos, there also was marked variability in Spanish language proficiency among U.S. neuropsychologists. It is interesting to note that there were very few differences in test use between neuropsychologists with high Spanish language proficiency compared with those with less proficiency in Spanish. However, there were marked differences in the use of translators. Neuropsychologists with less Spanish language proficiency used translators much more frequently than did neuropsychologists with greater language proficiency. They also used translators much more frequently when examining monolingual Spanish speakers as opposed to bilingual Spanish speakers. This finding makes sense, because without a translator, the monolingual English-speaking neuropsychologist would not be able to communicate with a monolingual Spanish-speaking patient. However, the use of translators is controversial, and many issues must be carefully evaluated and addressed (Ardila et al., 2002; Echemendia et al., 1997; Ponton & Ardila, 1999; Puente, Sol Mara, & Muñoz-Cespedes, 1997). Given the relationship between the need for services among Latinos and the limited number of Spanish-speaking neuropsychologists, the potential role of

translators is obvious. It remains critically important that these translators receive training in neuropsychological methods and practices to ensure the fidelity of their translations and the integrity of the test data.

The issue of test use and test development across cultures is also complex (Bracken & Barona, 1991; Echemendia et al., 2001; Geisinger, 1994; Harris, Echemendia, Ardila, & Rosselli, 2001; Reynolds & Kaiser, 1990; Van de Vijver & Hambleton, 1996). The data from this study document that bilingual Spanish speakers usually are given the English language version of a test, whereas monolingual Spanish speakers usually are given a translated version of the same test. Unfortunately, neuropsychologists are not reaching beyond what is most readily accessible. For example, although published Spanish language versions of some measures do exist and are available through international publishers, most practitioners still rely on their own verbatim translations. Generally, bilingual Spanish speakers are being treated as if they were English speakers. The effect of bilingualism on neuropsychological test performance remains an area in need of research, although there is a growing literature on cognitive models of bilingualism (cf. Kroll, Michael, & Sankaranaraynan, 1998). Ardila et al. (2002) addressed the levels of language proficiency exemplified within this group. At one end of the spectrum are English-dominant bilinguals who have relatively limited proficiency in Spanish; at the other end of the spectrum are Spanish-dominant bilinguals who have relatively diminished proficiency in English. Neuropsychological test performance may vary as a function of where an individual falls on this continuum. For example, Harris, Cullum, and Puente (1995) found no differences in scores when participants were tested in their dominant language on a verbal learning and memory task, but nonbalanced bilinguals learned fewer words and had lower retention compared with balanced bilinguals when tested in English as opposed to Spanish. Ardila et al. also pointed out that the language proficiency of the examiner is an important consideration because the examiner may not be equally proficient in Spanish and English. A mismatch between the patient's language abilities and those of the neuropsychologist may lead to errors in administration, interpretation, and diagnosis.

As noted earlier, although bilingual Spanish speakers were generally tested as though they were fluent English speakers, monolingual Spanish speakers usually were given a verbatim translation of an English language test. To a lesser extent, some monolingual Spanish speakers were given culturally adapted versions of a test. The difference between these two types of translations has a bearing on the validity of the test. Verbatim translations directly translate the English stimuli into Spanish. This type of translation is problematic because there are many words and phrases that cannot be translated directly (Bracken & Barona, 1991). Padilla (1979) argued that adaptation of a test to the new target culture is far superior to simple translation and back-translation. The process of adaptation requires that test items be changed and culturally adapted so that the new items accurately capture the meaning of the original items (Geisinger, 1994). Test translation also has been addressed by the International Test Commission (Van de Vijver & Hambleton, 1996) and by the *Standards for Educational and Psychological Testing* (American Educational Research Association, 1999). Each of these resources stresses the importance of demonstrating the reliability and validity of the adapted test with the new target group.

A common practice among neuropsychologists who evaluate monolingual Spanish speakers is to extemporaneously translate a test while testing the patient. Although this practice usually occurs because of necessity and frustration with the lack of formally developed tests, it is highly problematic. The "on-the-fly" nature of the translation does not allow for careful deliberation of the many variables involved in translating and adapting items; there is no back translation, there are no means to pilot and adjust the items, and there are no psychometric data that quantify the reliability and validity of the translation.

Once a test has been translated and the Latino has been tested, what reference norms should be used to interpret the test results? The results of this survey show that 67% of the time bilingual Spanish speakers are compared with English-speaking normative samples and monolingual Spanish speakers are compared with the same samples 23% of the time. The performance of monolingual Spanish speakers was compared using Latino norms 20% of the time and more often (57%) was not compared with norms at all; instead, the neuropsychologist chose to use clinical judgment. The use of clinical judgment rather than norms likely reflects neuropsychologists' perception that the use of English-speaking norms with monolingual Spanish speakers is inappropriate. Harris, Echemendia, Ardila, and Rosselli (2001) stated, "translating a test and using the normative tables from the original language version of the test, without documenting the comparability of norms is unacceptable" (p. 396). The consortium of the American Educational Research Association, the APA, and the National Council of Measurement in Education (American Educational Research Association, 1999)

also apply this standard to those for whom English is a second language. They also agree that norms generated primarily on English speakers should not be used for those people who learned English as a second language and who are not proficient in the language. If the norms are to be used, there must be some attempt to demonstrate the language proficiency of that individual.

The results of this survey provide some insight into the practices of U.S. neuropsychologists with Hispanic populations. The findings of this survey must be evaluated in light of the fact that the data were collected in 1994 and that they may or may not reflect current practices. Although we hope that practices have changed over the past 10 years, our experiences and those of our many colleagues suggest that these practices have not.

Conclusion

The United States is becoming increasingly diverse, and the Hispanic/Latino population is one of the fastest growing groups within this multicultural society. Latinos bring a rich culture to the United States and, as a group, are themselves highly heterogeneous. The results of this survey suggest that U.S. neuropsychologists are not prepared adequately to provide services to Latinos, nor do they have the appropriate tools to do so. Although there has been movement among test publishers in developing and norming tests in Spanish, much still has to be done. Test publishers often state that they do not provide Spanish language tests because they are not "marketable." The results of this survey indicate that, if available, U.S. neuropsychologists would use these tests. Given the demographic projections by the U.S. Bureau of the Census, it is likely that test publishers would profit from Spanish language tests if they adopted a long-range perspective. It is important that the major neuropsychology organizations (National Academy of Neuropsychology [NAN], APA Division 40, International Neuropsychological Society [INS]) work together to encourage test publishers to adapt existing tests and develop new measures for this population.

The issue of appropriate normative data is also critically important. Without the appropriate norms, the probability of misdiagnosis is unacceptably high. It is true that not only test publishers bear some of the responsibility for the lack of norms, but also the profession of neuropsychology and its members. U.S. neuropsychologists are providing services to a large number of Latinos. If organized, a subset of this group could work with each other to systematically collect normative data on the commonly used tests that have been identified in this survey. To accomplish this task, the professional organizations need to take a leadership role. We challenge NAN, APA Division 40, and INS, either collectively or individually, to provide the leadership and financial support that is necessary for such an endeavor.

References

American Educational Research Association. (1999). *Standards for educational and psychological testing.* Washington, DC: Author.

American Psychological Association. (1990). Guidelines for providers of psychological services to ethnic, linguistic, and culturally diverse populations. Washington, DC: Author.

American Psychological Association. (1992). Ethical principles of psychologists and code of conduct. *American Psychologist, 47,* 1597–1611.

American Psychological Association. (2002). Ethical principles and code of conduct. *American Psychologist, 57,* 1060–1073.

Ardila, A. (1998). Bilingualism: A neglected and chaotic area. *Aphasiology, 12,* 131–134.

Ardila, A., Rodriguez-Menendez, G., & Rosselli, M. (2002). Current issues in neuropsychological assessment with Hispanics/Latinos. In R. Ferraro (Ed.), *Minority and cross-cultural aspects of neuropsychological assessment* (pp. 161–179). Lisse, The Netherlands: Swets & Zeitlinger.

Bracken, B., & Barona, A. (1991). State of the art procedures for translating, validating, and using psychoeducational tests in cross-cultural assessment. *School Psychology International, 12,* 119–132.

Butler, M., Retzlaff, P., & Vanderploeg, R. (1991). Neuropsychological test usage. *Professional Psychology: Research and Practice, 22,* 510–512.

Cuellar, I. (1998). Cross-cultural clinical psychological assessment of Hispanic Americans. *Journal of Personality Assessment, 70,* 71–86.

Dalpon, H., & Tighe, P. (1996). *Idea Proficiency Test.* Brea, CA: Ballard & Tighe Publishers.

Duncan, S. E., & DeAvila, E. A. (1990). *Language Assessment Scale.* Monterey, CA: CTB/McGraw-Hill.

Echemendia, R. J., & Julian, L. (2002). Neuropsychological assessment of Latino children. In R. Ferraro (Ed.), *Minority and cross-cultural aspects of neuropsychological assessment* (pp. 181–203). Lisse, The Netherlands: Swets & Zeitlinger.

Echemendia, R. J., Harris, J. G., Congett, S. M., Diaz, L. M., & Puente, A. (1997). Neuropsychological training and practices with Hispanics: A national survey. *Clinical neuropsychologist, 11,* 229–243.

Geisinger, K. (1994). Cross-cultural normative assessment: Translation and adaptation issues influencing the normative interpretation of assessment instruments. *Psychological Assessment, 6,* 304–312.

Harcourt Educational Measurement. (2002). *Stanford English Language Proficiency Test.* San Antonio, TX: Harcourt.

Harris, J. G., Cullum, C. M., & Puente, A. (1995). Effects of bilingualism on verbal learning and memory in Hispanic adults. *Journal of the International Neuropsychological Society, 1,* 10–16.

Harris, J. G., Echemendia, R. J., Ardila, A., & Rosselli, M. (2001). Cross-cultural cognitive and neuropsychological assessment. In H. J. J. Andrews & D. Saklofske (Eds.), *Handbook of psychoeducational assessment* (pp. 392–414). San Diego, CA: Academic.

Harris, J. G., Tulsky, D. S., & Schultheis, M. T. (2003). Assessment of the non-native English speaker: Assimilating history and research findings to guide clinical practice. In D. Tulsky, G. Chelune, R. Ivnik, A. Prifitera, D. Saklofske, R. Heaton, R. Bornstein, & M. Zedbetter (Eds.). *Clinical interpretation of the WAIS–III and WMS–III* (pp. 343–390). San Diego, CA: Academic.

Kroll, J., Michael, E., & Sankaranaraynan, A. (1998). A model of bilingual representation and its implications for second language acquisition. In A. F. Healy & L. E. Bourne, Jr. (Eds.), *Foreign language learning: Psycholinguistic studies on training and retention* (pp. 365–395). Mahwah, NJ: Lawrence Erlbaum Associates, Inc.

Melendez, F. (1994). The Spanish version of the WAIS: Some ethical considerations. *The Clinical Neuropsychologist, 8,* 388–393.

Padilla, A. M. (1979). Cultural factors in testing of Hispanic Americans: A review and some suggestions of the future. In R. W. T. S. H. White (Ed.), *Testing, teaching and learning: Report of a conference on testing.* Washington, DC: National Institute of Education.

Ponton, M., & Ardila, A. (1999). The future of neuropsychology with Hispanic populations in the United States. *Archives of Clinical Neuropsychology, 14,* 565–580.

Puente, A. E., Sol Mora, M., & Muñoz-Cespedes, J. M. (1997). Neuropsychological assessment of Spanish-speaking children and youth. In C. R. Reynolds & E. Fletcher-Janzen (Eds.), *Handbook of clinical child neuropsychology* (2nd. ed., pp. 371–383). New York: Plenum.

Reynolds, C. R., & Kaiser, S. M. (1990). Test bias in psychological assessment. In T. B. G. C. R. Reynolds (Eds.), *The handbook of school psychology* (2nd. ed., pp. 487–525). New York: Wiley.

U.S. Bureau of the Census. (2000). Population estimate. Retrieved January 10, 2004, from http://www.census.gov

Van de Vijver, F., & Hambleton, R. K. (1996). Translating tests: Some practical guidelines. *European Psychologist, 1,* 89–99.

Woodcock, R. W., & Muñoz-Sandoval, A. F. (1993). *Woodcock-Muñoz Language Survey.* Itasca, IL: Riverside.

Applied Neuropsychology
2004, Vol. 11, No. 1, 13–22

Racial and Ethnic Diversity Among Trainees and Professionals in Psychology and Neuropsychology: Needs, Trends, and Challenges

Felicia Hill-Briggs

Department of Physical Medicine and Rehabilitation, Johns Hopkins School of Medicine, Baltimore, Maryland, USA

Jovier D. Evans

Department of Psychology, Indiana University Purdue University Indianapolis, Indianapolis, Indiana, USA

Marc A. Norman

Department of Psychiatry, University of California, San Diego, California, USA

The United States is rapidly becoming a more racially and ethnically diverse nation, bringing the challenge of ensuring that health care specialties, including neuropsychology, are representative of and competent to serve the needs of this population. Initiatives have been undertaken to increase minority representation in training for psychology and neuropsychology. However, tracking progress requires reliable race/ethnicity data collection and reporting. On the 2002 American Psychological Association (APA) Directory Survey (APA Research Office, 2002), up to 42% of the APA membership and up to 25% of the Division 40 membership did not specify race/ethnicity status. Within Division 40, data for members who did report race/ethnicity suggest that representation of Hispanic, Asian, Black/African American, and Native American members lags substantially behind that of White members. Improved methods for collecting information on race/ethnicity are needed to meet diversity objectives.

Key words: minority, professional issues, training, professional membership, demographics, psychology

The United States is becoming a more racially and ethnically diverse nation, with rapid increases in minority populations over the past 2 decades. From 1980 to 2000, the White[1] population decreased from 83.1% to 75.1%. In contrast, the Hispanic population increased from 6.4% to 12.5%, the Black population increased from 11.7% to 12.3%, the Asian and Pacific Islander population increased from 1.5% to 3.7%, and the American Indian and Alaskan Native population increased from 0.6% to 0.9% (U.S. Bureau of the Census, 2000). Census data estimate that by the year 2055, the United States will be a fully pluralistic nation, with no one racial or ethnic group in the majority. These changing demographics bring the challenge of ensuring that health care specialties, including neuropsychology, are representative of and competent to serve the needs of this pluralistic population.

The purpose of this article is threefold: (a) to identify, in light of the changing demographics of the U.S. population, the rationale for increasing diversity among trainees and professionals within the health care workforce and the implications of these identified needs for neuropsychology; (b) to identify initiatives to increase representation of racial/ethnic minorities

---

[1]The terms used in the text to refer to the racial/ethnic groups discussed are *White, Black/African American, Hispanic, Asian,* and *Native American.* However, other terms are used when presenting information from sources, including the U.S. Bureau of the Census, the American Psychological Association Research Office, and the Association of American Medical Colleges, because each source uses different terminology in its collecting and reporting of data on race/ethnicity. When reporting data from such sources, the actual terminology or categories used by those agencies or organizations is used (e.g., *Black, Latino[a], Hispanic/Latino[a], American Indian, Asian/Pacific Islander*).

Requests for reprints should be sent to Felicia Hill-Briggs, Department of Physical Medicine and Rehabilitation, Meyer 1–164, 600 North Wolfe Street, Baltimore, MD 21287, USA. E-mail: fbriggsh@jhmi.edu

13

within psychology and within neuropsychology as a subfield; and (c) to examine data on progress toward increased diversity among trainees and professionals in psychology and neuropsychology. In compiling data on progress in minority representation in psychology and neuropsychology, limitations were identified in the status of race and ethnicity data reporting and collection in psychology and neuropsychology. The Discussion section focuses on the challenge of creating systematic procedures for race and ethnicity data collection in the field to analyze and interpret the status of diversity within the training and professions of psychology and neuropsychology.

Rationale for Increasing Diversity Among Health Care Providers

The need for diversity among physicians and other health care providers has received a great deal of attention in light of federal recommendations and profession-initiated efforts to meet the challenge of an increasingly diverse population (Barzansky, Jonas, & Etzel, 2000; Kavanagh & Kennedy, 1992). Cohen, Gabriel, and Terrell (2002) asserted a rationale for the need for systematic initiatives to increase minority representation among health care providers, not only in the physician workforce, but also in other health professions that have not achieved "optimal diversity":

> Putting aside issues of equity and fairness for the moment, at least four practical reasons can be put forth for attaining greater diversity in the health care workforce: (1) advancing cultural competency, (2) increasing access to high-quality health care services, (3) strengthening the medical research agenda, and (4) ensuring optimal management of the health care system …
>
> Recruitment of these persons into the educational pipeline of the health professions is, of course, what determines not only their ultimate representation in the workforce but also their influence on the educational process itself. (pp. 91–92)

Cultural competency and care of underserved populations are two concerns that have come to the forefront in the dialogue regarding minority representation among health care professionals (Kavanagh & Kennedy, 1992). The increased representation of ethnic minorities in the population and, consequently, in persons served by health professionals mandates that professionals become culturally competent to provide effective care (Smedley, Stith, & Nelson, 2003). In training providers to become culturally competent, curricula err in reducing ethnic and cultural education to learning of typologies or stereotypes for each racial/ethnic group (Smedley et al., 2003). To achieve cultural competence, trainees and professionals need not only textbook knowledge and curricula, but also experiences within a diverse academic environment analogous to the diversity of the society and environment in which they will be expected to practice (Cohen et al., 2002; Kavanagh & Kennedy, 1992).

The contribution of ethnic minority health care professionals to the care of underserved populations has particular import. Data on professional practices reveal that, compared with White physicians, for example, African American, Hispanic American, and Native American physicians are significantly more likely to provide care to underserved and uninsured populations that are vulnerable to disparities in health care access and quality and to provide care within ethnic minority communities (Cantor, Miles, Baker, & Barker, 1996; Komaromy et al., 1996). In addition, patients tend to choose health care providers who are similar to themselves in race/ethnicity (Saha, Taggart, Komaromy, & Bindman, 2000), and racial/ethnic concordance between patient and provider is directly associated with increased patient satisfaction (Cooper-Patrick et al., 1999; Saha, Komaromy, Koepsell, & Bindman, 1999). Sociocultural differences between patient and provider that are not adequately addressed result in poor satisfaction, poor adherence, poorer outcomes, and racial/ethnic disparities in care (Cooper-Patrick et al., 1999; Langer, 1999; Morales, Cunningham, Brown, Liu, & Hays, 1999). Moreover, language discordance between patient and provider serves as a significant barrier to health care communication, quality, effectiveness, and patient satisfaction among the nearly 14 million persons living in the United States who have no or limited English language skills (Smedley et al., 2003).

Several findings regarding the need for increased representation among health care providers for reduction of health disparities (Smedley et al., 2003) have direct impact on the practice of psychology and neuropsychology. First, among the medical conditions noted as having high disparities in health care quality, services, and outcomes for minorities are conditions for which neuropsychology is often involved, including stroke, HIV/AIDS, and organ transplantation. Second, empirical research and federal reports have documented that mental health services, more than other areas of health and medicine, have been found to be plagued by disparities in service availability and access to racially and culturally diverse groups, which results in greater disability among racial and ethnic minorities (Smedley et al., 2003). Third, in addition to health disparities caused by access and availability, the National Institutes of Health and the Institute of Medicine (Smedley et al., 2003) emphasized the need for research focused on each ethnic group to identify personal (e.g., cognitive, emotional, behavioral), societal, and interpersonal (e.g., social support, patient–provider relationships) factors that also contribute to health disparities. Finally, with regard to providing services to non-English or limited English speakers, the U.S. Department of Health and Human Services Standards for Culturally and Linguistically Appropriate Services (U.S. Department of Health and Human Services, 2000) mandated that health care organizations provide competent language assistance or intervention by bilingual staff or interpreters and that the practice of using family and friends to provide interpretation services is detrimental to trust in health care and to patient confidentiality, except on explicit request by the patient (Smedley et al., 2003). Psychology and neuropsychology must meet the challenge of providing culturally competent clinical services, training, and research that address the needs and current disparities of a multiethnic and multilingual society.

Strategic Initiatives Toward Increasing Diversity in Psychology and Neuropsychology

The American Psychological Association (APA), APA Division 40, and the National Academy of Neuropsychology (NAN) have undertaken strategic initiatives to address needs for diversity within the field. In response to an APA resolution identifying recruitment, retention, and training of minorities as one of the organization's highest priorities, in 1994, the APA Commission on Ethnic Minority Recruitment, Retention, and Training in Psychology was established. The commission's recommendations focused on several objectives: (a) the transformation of education in psychology from the high school through postdoctoral and continuing education levels in ways that would significantly increase (from the 5%–6% at the time) the proportion of psychologists who were racial/ethnic minorities; (b) the demonstration, by all psychologists, of at least minimal competence in multicultural training, research,

and practice issues; and (c) the demonstration of valuing diversity within academic settings and the enhancement of the educational and departmental environment to promote retention of ethnic minority faculty and students (Commision on Ethnic Minority Recruitment, Retention, and Training in Psychology, 1997).

Consistent with the APA's *Guidelines on Multicultural Education, Training, Research, Practice, and Organizational Change for Psychologists* (APA, 2003), the mission of the Division 40 Ethnic Minority Affairs Committee (Div40 EMA) is to promote the integration of diverse populations into the fabric of neuropsychological practice, research, teaching, and training to provide neuropsychologists with the knowledge and resources to better understand and serve an increasingly diverse U.S. population and to reduce the historic inequities present in the field of neuropsychology. The specific diverse populations targeted by this committee include those who have been historically marginalized or disenfranchised within and by neuropsychology on the basis of their racial/ethnic heritage and social group identity or membership (APA, 2003), including African Americans, Asian Americans, Hispanic Americans, Native Americans, and other biracial/ multiethnic, multiracial groups.

As such, this committee has three overarching objectives. The first objective is to promote the provision of culturally competent neuropsychological services to persons of color by increasing awareness and providing training opportunities on cross-cultural/multicultural assessment issues among all neuropsychologists. The second objective is to stimulate the highest quality of neuropsychological research among minority populations by increasing awareness for the need for such research among the neuropsychological community, as well as by providing research resources and facilitating consultation and mentoring on cross-cultural/multicultural research-related issues. The final overarching objective of this committee is to strongly encourage the career development of neuropsychologists with diverse ethnic or racial backgrounds, as the infusion of increasing numbers of competent neuropsychologists will likely broaden the field's conceptualization and implementation of practice, research, and training. The Div40 EMA committee has established an e-mail listserv to promote dialogue among its constituents, has published its mission statement on the Division 40 Web site, and is establishing a mentoring program to foster more collaborative efforts with senior neuropsychologists in the fields of clinical research and practice.

Among the objectives of NAN are to provide advancement and information resources for scientific brain–behavior relationships, as well as to provide guidelines for standards of practice, training development, and support for student involvement. To promote these goals within the context of ethnic groups and individual differences, the NAN Cultural and Diversity Committee was created. A primary effort of this committee has been the translation of educational materials into other languages that will be available through the NAN Web site. The committee also is working on initiatives with APA Division 40 to analyze and increase minority participation in neuropsychology by creating and promoting mentorship opportunities for all levels of clinical practice and research. The committee is particularly interested in increasing ethnic minority graduate student involvement in neuropsychology and developing approaches that will enhance the cultural training of all neuropsychologists.

Tracking Progress on Initiatives to Increase Diversity Within Psychology and Neuropsychology

Sources of Information on Race and Ethnicity

To examine the current status of racial and ethnic minority representation in psychology and neuropsychology, information on the number and percentage of persons within training programs and professional memberships, by race/ethnicity, were solicited from APA, APA Division 40 Clinical Neuropsychology, NAN, Association of Psychology Postdoctoral and Internship Centers (APPIC), and Association of Postdoctoral Programs in Clinical Neuropsychology (APPCN). Within the professional organizations (APA and NAN), although race, ethnicity, and gender are demographic characteristics listed in membership applications, these fields are voluntary and are, therefore, subject to high nonresponse rates. Race and ethnicity data are not requested in APPIC or APPCN applications for trainees.

The APA Research Office served as a primary source for information reported in this article on race and ethnicity in psychology training and professional memberships. The APA Research Office conducts periodic surveys via mail to collect data, including characteristics of students in doctoral and master's degree departments of psychology (i.e., the biennial Characteristics of Graduate Departments of Psychology Survey), em-

ployment status of new doctorates in psychology (i.e., the biennial Doctorate Employment Survey), and characteristics of the APA membership (i.e., the annual APA Directory Survey).

Racial and Ethnic Representation in Psychology Training

Trends in percentages of nonminorities and minorities completing training in psychology are available for the years 1976 through 2001, based on data gathered from APA Research Office surveys (Fennel & Kohout, 2002); compilations (APA Research Office, 2003); and data compiled by the Commission on Ethnic Minority Recruitment, Retention, and Training in Psychology (1997). Figure 1 presents data available on percentages of racial/ethnic minorities in each level of psychology education (relative to the total persons in each level of psychology education), including persons completing the bachelor's degree in psychology, persons enrolled in graduate programs in psychology, persons completing the master's degree, and persons completing the doctoral degree. Data points are shown for the years reported by the different sources from which data were drawn. Data reveal a pattern of increases in minority representation across all levels of training. In 2000, the percentage of ethnic minorities who completed a bachelor of arts degree, who were enrolled in graduate training, and who completed a doctorate degree each remained below 30%, which is the percentage of ethnic minorities within the general population (U.S. Bureau of the Census, 2000).

With regard to percentages of students representing different race/ethnicity groups, in the year 1999–2000, of the 9,576 full-time doctoral students enrolled in U.S. graduate psychology departments, 6,851 (72%) were White, 879 (9%) were Hispanic, 693 (7%) were African American, 398 (4%) were Asian American, 83 (< 1%) were American Indian/Alaska Native, and 114 (1%) were multiple ethnicities (Fennell & Kohout, 2002). The authors of this report cautioned that these findings were based on the reporting of 100 departments that responded to the 2000–2001 survey. Therefore, the data were described as undercounting actual numbers of students enrolled (Fennell & Kohout, 2002).

Data on racial/ethnic minority applicants to internships in psychology are available for the year 2001–2002 (Pate, 2001). A total of 293 programs were included in the data analysis from a 76% response yield of doctoral departments surveyed. Of 2,357 known students seeking

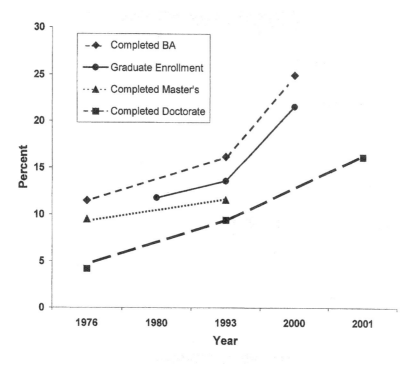

Figure 1. Percentage of racial/ethnic minority students at four levels of psychology training. Levels of training represented are as follows: (a) persons who completed a bachelor of arts (BA) degree in psychology, (b) persons who were enrolled in a graduate program in psychology, (c) persons who completed a master's degree in psychology, and (d) persons who completed a doctoral degree in psychology for selected years from 1976 through 2001. Data points for levels of training vary by year because of differences in reporting by the sources from which data were compiled.

internships for the year 2001–2002, 1,980 (84%) were not minorities, and 377 (16%) were minorities.

Ethnic and Racial Representation in Neuropsychology Training

Doctorate degrees in clinical neuropsychology as a subfield represented 2% of all new doctorates in psychology in 2001, while clinical psychology, as a separate subfield, represented 35% of all new doctorates (APA Research Office, 2001). No data are currently available on percentages of racial/ethnic minority persons completing doctorate degrees in neuropsychology, seeking internships in neuropsychology, or seeking postdoctoral fellowships/ residency programs in neuropsychology. Because neuropsychology represents only 2% of doctoral degrees in psychology, the numbers of ethnic minorities receiving doctoral degrees in neuropsychology is likely quite small and deserves study. APPCN may be a source through which data on racial/ethnic representation in neuropsychology subfield training can be researched in the future.

Ethnic and Racial Representation in APA and Division 40 Clinical Neuropsychology Memberships

The 2002 APA Directory Survey (APA Research Office) provided membership data for APA and for APA Division 40 by racial/ethnic group. In 2002, there were 93,406 members of APA and 4,184 members of Division 40, inclusive of all membership categories. Of total members in APA specifying race/ethnicity status ($N = 67,653$), minorities numbered 4,875 (7.2%), and of total members of Division 40 specifying race/ethnicity status ($N = 3,603$), minorities numbered 244 (6.8%). Percentages of nonminority and minority members of APA and Division 40, by racial/ethnic category, are shown for membership status categories of member (Figure 2), associate (Figure 3), and fellow (Figure 4). Of significance, race/ethnicity was not specified for large percentages of the APA and the Division 40 membership, especially for APA associates (43%), Division 40 associates (25%), and APA members (25%). As a result, conclusions are not easily drawn because it is unknown how many of those not specifying race/ethnicity might have increased the

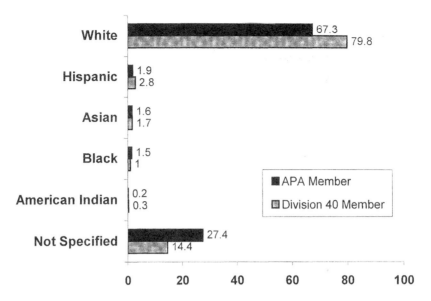

Figure 2. Race/ethnicity of APA members and Division 40 Clinical Neuropsychology members holding member status in 2002. APA member status N = 80,583; Division 40 member status N = 3,829. Source is 2002 APA Directory Survey (APA Research Office, 2002).

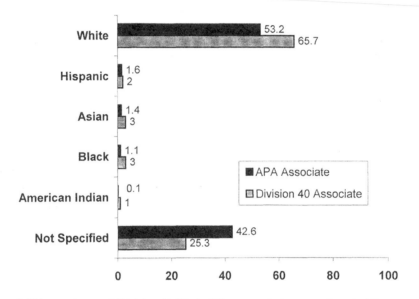

Figure 3. Race/ethnicity of APA members and Division 40 Clinical Neuropsychology members holding associate membership status in 2002. APA associate N = 8,108; Division 40 associate N = 99. Source is 2002 APA Directory Survey (APA Research Office, 2002).

percentages of minorities shown. However, of those who did indicate race/ethnicity, the very low percentages of minorities (ranging from 0.1% to 1.7%) across ethnic groups for both APA and Division 40 suggests that minority representation may lag substantially behind that of nonminority membership.

Comparison of two recent years of Division 40 membership data on race and ethnicity suggests relative stability in percentages of members who reported belonging to each of the race/ethnicity categories (see Figure 5; APA Research Office, 2000, 2002). The number of persons not specifying race or ethnicity, however, increased somewhat in 2002 (14%) compared with 2000 (10%).

Discussion

Collectively, APA, Division 40, and NAN have put forth mission statements and have instituted strategic initiatives to increase the diversity and cultural competence of psychologists and neuropsychologists to prepare them to meet the needs of a growing multiethnic U.S. national population. Data reported suggest that progress is being made toward increasing representation of ethnic minorities within the training programs in psychology, both at the undergraduate and graduate levels. However, data on ethnic minority representation in neuropsychology training are not currently available.

18

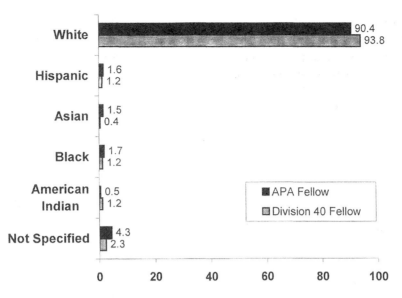

Figure 4.   Race/ethnicity of APA members and Division 40 Clinical Neuropsychology members holding fellow membership status in 2002. APA fellow N = 4,715; Division 40 fellow N = 256. Source is 2002 APA Directory Survey (APA Research Office, 2002).

Moreover, data on race and ethnicity in APA and Division 40 professional memberships suggest low numbers of minority representation, but these data must be interpreted with caution because of high rates of nonspecification of race or ethnicity status.

To analyze the effectiveness of initiatives toward increasing ethnic minority representation in psychology and neuropsychology, a primary challenge to the field is the establishment of processes to increase the report-

ing and collection of data. In this article, sensitivity to reporting race/ethnicity data was evident. For example, in the 2002 APA Directory Survey (APA, 2002), persons not specifying race/ethnicity reached as high as 43% in some membership categories. In contrast, persons not specifying gender for membership status categories in APA ranged from 0% to 1.6% (0.5% for total APA membership); in Division 40, nonspecification of gender ranged from 0% to 0.1% (0% for total Division

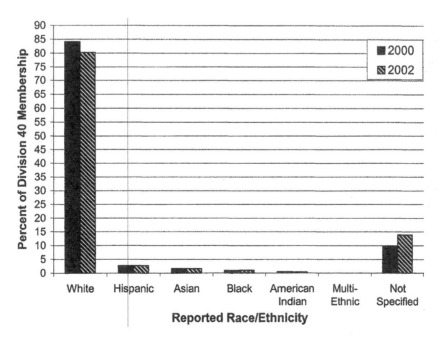

Figure 5.   Reported race/ethnicity of Division 40 total membership for the years 2000 and 2002. Division 40 total membership in 2000, N = 4,067. Division 40 total membership in 2002, N = 4,184. Category Multi-Ethnic includes persons responding to Multi-Ethnic or Other. Figure adapted from APA Research Office data ("Reported Race/Ethnicity of Division 40 Total Membership, 2000 and 2002"). Copyright © 2000 and 2002 by the American Psychological Association. Adapted with permission.

40 membership). Sensitivity to collecting data on race/ethnicity also was apparent. Race/ethnicity is not included on applications completed by students for APPIC or APPCN. Moreover, listing race and ethnicity as voluntary fields in professional membership applications makes them subject to high nonresponse rates. The APA Research Office has served a critical role in conducting surveys to analyze data by race/ethnicity; however, the data are based on response rates to the mailed survey format and can be subject to under-representation of actual numbers (Fennell & Kohout, 2002).

Reasons for the sensitivity to reporting of data on race/ethnicity include issues of privacy and confidentiality from the agency/organization perspective, personal preference not to disclose, need for protection against bias, and potential resulting legal and political issues (Smedley et al., 2003). However, to address issues of diversity in professional training and practice and to monitor effectiveness of initiatives to promote diversity, collecting these data is essential (Cohen, 2003; Perez, 2003). As the field of psychology faces the challenge of race/ethnicity data collection, federal and legal practices and guidelines and effective strategies within the medical field may serve as guides for consideration.

Federal and Legal Policies and Recommendations Regarding Collection of Data on Race, Ethnicity, and Primary Language in Health Care Settings

The Institute of Medicine (Smedley et al., 2003) discussed findings from a report of the extent to which reporting of race, ethnicity, and primary language are mandated or encouraged by federal policies and an analysis of how current law regarding reporting/data collection is understood, interpreted, and implemented by federal agencies. The report analyzed regulations; statutes; federal agency policies; and practices related to race, ethnicity, and primary language in health care settings. Three primary conclusions from the report, which are supported by precedent and research (Perez, 2003), are that (a) the collection of data on race, ethnicity, and primary language is legal and authorized under Title VI of the Civil Rights Act of 1964; (b) many federal policies emphasize the need for the collection of race, ethnicity, and primary language data; and (c) without collecting such data, it is impossible to measure success of efforts toward federal goals of eliminating health disparities. The Health Insurance Portability and Accountability Act (HIPAA) provides an example,

however, of the failure of systematic implementation of mandatory reporting even in federal policies, despite consensus among federal and legal agencies. The finding that race/ethnicity is not a required code in HIPAA led to a specific recommendation to revise standards for implementing HIPAA to designate the race and ethnicity data code as mandatory for claims and enrollment (Smedley et al., 2003).

Examples of Effective Practices Regarding Collection of Data on Race and Ethnicity in Medicine

Within the field of medicine, strategic initiatives to increase diversity among physicians have been substantial, and methods for reporting data on race and ethnicity have been effective. The Association of American Medical Colleges (AAMC), a nonprofit association of all U.S.-accredited medical schools and major teaching hospitals, reports data on characteristics of medical school students and residents as early as 1950 through the present (Cohen, 2003). In addition to AAMC, 100% response rates are reported consistently to surveys from sources including the Medical Education Research and Information Database of the APA and the Liaison Committee on Medical Education Annual Medical School Questionnaire, resulting in confidence that accurate numbers regarding race and ethnicity have been captured (e.g., Barzansky, Jonas, & Etzel, 2000; Kwakwa & Jonasson, 1999). As an example, in 1990, with implementation of the AAMC "Project 3000 by 2000," a large-scale, multifaceted, affirmative initiative to double the number of underrepresented minorities admitted each year to medical schools (Nickens et al., 1994), a sharp increase in minority admissions to medical schools could be tracked effectively and analyzed against historical data (Cohen et al., 2002). The increase in diversity followed a 15-year period of relative stagnation in minority matriculates. Data revealed that in 1999, the physician workforce consisted of 9.1% Asians and Pacific Islanders (combined category), 3.5% Hispanics, 2.6% African Americans, and 0.1% Native Americans (Cohen et al., 2002). Systematic data collection also has resulted in the ability to analyze race, ethnicity, and gender representation within medical specialties, including orthopedics (e.g., Ayers, 1999; England & Pierce, 1999), family practice (e.g., Lewis-Stevenson, Hueston, Mainous, Bazell, & Ye, 2001), and surgery (e.g., American College of Surgeons, 1994; Kwakwa & Jonasson, 1996, 1999).

Implications for Psychology and Neuropsychology and Future Directions

The strategic initiatives undertaken to increase racial/ethnic minority representation in psychology and neuropsychology necessitate careful efforts to increase data collection and monitoring of progress. Indeed, improvement in the data collection and reporting of race and ethnicity may be a necessary first step in attaining diversity goals. Efforts within the field of medicine with regard to race and ethnicity data collection and reporting may serve as a model on which the field of psychology can build. Clear commitment of the profession of psychology to identified diversity initiatives and strong communication regarding this commitment are critical for achieving cooperation in race and ethnicity data collection within the field. To increase the effectiveness of the current system of voluntary identification (or nonidentification) of race/ethnicity status, efforts to increase dissemination of information about the use of such data and the importance of reporting such data for APA research and initiatives are warranted. Furthermore, inquiry regarding APA member reluctance to report demographic data and attitudes/beliefs associated with identifying race/ethnicity status would prove beneficial. Results of such inquiry may prove enlightening not only in devising the means to increase reporting, but also for examining issues of sensitivity and stigma associated with discussion of race and ethnicity within the profession.

Further steps can be taken toward increasing racial and ethnic diversity within the subspecialty of neuropsychology. Initiatives can focus on increasing knowledge and understanding of neuropsychology as a profession among students entering the psychology pipeline. Such efforts might include using existing minority neuropsychology graduate students to speak at universities with large minority populations and providing funding for minority neuropsychologists to visit programs and provide education about the profession and the course of training. Moreover, continued growth of research addressing multicultural issues in neuropsychology can be fostered. A recommended initiative is research awards or recognition for neuropsychological publications or conference presentations that contribute to greater understanding of or improved service delivery to diverse groups.

Finally, this article focused on traditional cultural groups (e.g., race/ethnicity). For psychology to address the needs of a truly diverse society, other groups and cultures, such as those based on gender, sexual orientation, and disability, must be the focus of strategic efforts toward both multicultural education and representation.

References

American College of Surgeons. (1994). *Longitudinal study of surgical residents: 1992–1993.* Chicago: Education and Surgical Services Department of the American College of Surgeons.

American Psychological Association. (2003). Guidelines on multicultural education, training, research, practice, and organizational change for psychologists. *American Psychologist, 58,* 377–402.

American Psychological Association Research Office. (2000). *2000 APA directory survey.* Washington, DC: Author.

American Psychological Association Research Office. (2002). *2002 APA directory survey.* Washington, DC: Author.

American Psychological Association Research Office. (2001). *PhD graduates by subfield of degree: 2001.* Washington, DC: Author.

American Psychological Association Research Office. (2003). *Where are new psychologists going? Employment, debt, and salary data.* Paper presented at the annual convention of the Western Psychological Association, Vancouver, British Columbia. Retrieved July 21, 2003, from http://research@apa.org

Ayers, C. E. (1999). Minorities and the orthopaedic profession. *Clinical Orthopaedics and Related Research, 362,* 58–64.

Barzansky, B., Jonas, H. S., & Etzel, S. I. (2000). Educational programs in U.S. medical schools, 1999–2000. *Journal of the American Medical Association, 284,* 1114–1120.

Cantor, J. C., Miles, E. L., Baker, L. C., & Barker, D. C. (1996). Physician service to the uninsured: Implications for affirmative action in medical education. *Inquiry, 33,* 167–180.

Cohen, J. J. (2003). The consequences of premature abandonment of affirmative action in medical school admissions. *Journal of the American Medical Association, 289,* 1143–1149.

Cohen, J. J., Gabriel, B. A., & Terrell, C. (2002). The case for diversity in the health care workforce. *Health Affairs, 21,* 90–102.

Commission on Ethnic Minority Recruitment, Retention, and Training in Psychology. (1997). *Visions and transformations...The final report.* Washington, DC: Author.

Cooper-Patrick, L., Gallo, J. J., Gonzales, J. J., Vu, H. T., Powe, N. R., Nelson, C., et al. (1999). Race, gender, and partnership in the patient–physician relationship. *Journal of the American Medical Association, 282,* 583–589.

England, S. P., & Pierce, R. O. (1999). Current diversity in orthopaedics. *Clinical Orthopaedics and Related Research, 362,* 40–43.

Fennell, K., & Kohout, J. (2002). *Characteristics of graduate departments of psychology: 1999–2000.* Washington, DC: APA Research Office.

Grieco, E. M., & Cassidy, R. C. (2001). Overview of race and Hispanic origin: Census 200 brief. Retrieved July 14, 2003, from http://www.census.gov

Kavanagh, K. H., & Kennedy, P. H. (1992). *Promoting cultural diversity: Strategies for health care professionals.* Newbury Park, CA: Sage.

Komaromy, M., Grumbach, K., Drake, M., Vranizan, K., Lurie, N., Keane, D., et al. (1996). The role of Black and Hispanic physicians in providing health care for underserved populations. *New England Journal of Medicine, 334,* 1305–1310.

Kwakwa, F., & Jonasson, O. (1996). The longitudinal study of surgical residents, 1993–1994. *Journal of the American College of Surgeons, 183,* 425–433.

Kwakwa, F., & Jonasson, O. (1999). The longitudinal study of surgical residents, 1994–1996. *Journal of the American College of Surgeons, 188,* 575–585.

Langer, N. (1999). Culturally competent professionals in therapeutic alliances enhance patient compliance. *Journal of Health Care for the Poor and Underserved, 10,* 19–26.

Lewis-Stevenson, S., Hueston, W. J., Mainous, A. G., Bazell, P. C., & Ye, X. (2001). Female and underrepresented minority faculty in academic departments of family medicine: Are women and minorities better off in family medicine? *Family Medicine, 33,* 459–465.

Morales, L. S., Cunningham, W. E., Brown, J. A., Liu, H., & Hays, R. D. (1999). Are Latinos less satisfied with communication by health care providers? *Journal of General Internal Medicine, 14,* 409–417.

Nickens, H. W., Ready, T., & Petersdorf, R. G. (1994). Project 3000 by 2000—racial and ethnic diversity in US medical schools. *New England Journal of Medicine, 331,* 472–476.

Pate, W. (2001). *2000 demand for predoctoral internship survey.* Washington, DC: APA Research Office.

Petersdorf, R. G. (1994). Project 3000 by 2000—racial and ethnic diversity in US medical schools. *New England Journal of Medicine, 331,* 472–476.

Perez, T. E. (2003). The civil rights dimension of racial and ethnic disparities in health status. In B. D. Smedley, A. Y. Stith, & A. R. Nelson (Eds.). *Unequal treatment: Confronting racial and ethnic disparities in health care* (pp. 626–663). Washington, DC: National Academy Press.

Saha, S., Komaromy, M., Koepsell, T. D., & Bindman, A. B. (1999). Patient–physician racial concordance and the perceived quality and use of health care. *Archives of Internal Medicine, 159,* 997–1004.

Saha, S., Taggart, S. H., Komaromy, M., & Bindman, A. B. (2000). Do patients choose physicians of their own race? *Health Affairs, 19,* 76–83.

Smedley, B. D., Stith, A. Y., & Nelson, A. R. (Eds.). (2003). *Unequal treatment: Confronting racial and ethnic disparities in health care.* Washington, DC: National Academy Press.

U.S. Bureau of the Census. (2002). United States—Race and Hispanic origin: 1790 to 1990. Retrieved July 14, 2003, from http://www.census.gov

U.S. Department of Health and Human Services, Office of Minority Health. (2000). Culturally and linguistically appropriate services in health care. Final Report. 65 Fed. Reg. 80865–80879 (Dec. 22, 2000).

Applied Neuropsychology
2004, Vol. 11, No. 1, 23–36

Neuropsychological Assessment of Asian Americans: Demographic Factors, Cultural Diversity, and Practical Guidelines

Tony M. Wong

*Department of Physical Medicine and Rehabilitation, University of Rochester School of
Medicine & Dentistry, Rochester, New York, USA*

Daryl E. Fujii

Hawaii State Hospital, Honolulu, Hawaii, USA

*Asian Americans belong to 1 of the most rapidly growing ethnic minority groups in the United
States. Clinical neuropsychologists unfamiliar with Asian American peoples and cultures may
not be able to perform an adequate evaluation with an individual of Asian descent because of
lack of understanding of how cultural variables might affect the assessment. This article at-
tempts to provide some basic knowledge and principles by which to guide neuropsychologists
who might work with an Asian American patient by (a) familiarizing the reader with basic information and descriptions of some of the major specific Asian subgroups, (b) providing a context within which neuropsychological test selection and interpretation can be adjusted to account for cultural and linguistic factors, and (c) providing practical suggestions for working
with Asian American clients in a neuropsychological setting.*

Key words: neuropsychological assessment, Asian American, cultural diversity, cultural variables

A growing literature addressing the need to examine
cross-cultural factors in neuropsychological assessment (e.g., Ardila, 1995; Ardila, Rosselli, & Puente,
1994; Nell, 2000; Wong, Strickland, Fletcher-Janzen,
Ardila, & Reynolds, 2000) has emerged recently. This
has been a critical development, because as the ethnic
diversity of the U.S. population continues to grow,
more situations will occur in which a clinical neuropsychologist will be asked to evaluate a patient or client
whose cultural/ethnic background might be different
from or unfamiliar to the professional's. Unless the
neuropsychologist has minimal, adequate knowledge
of how the patient's background might influence the assessment process and results, a valid evaluation is pre-
cluded. This article focuses on issues related to the neuropsychological assessment of Asian Americans, one
of the most rapidly growing ethnic-minority groups in
the United States.

The U.S. Bureau of the Census uses the term *Asian*
to refer to people having origins in any of the peoples of
the Far East, Southeast Asia, or the Indian subcontinent
(Barnes & Bennett, 2002). Thus, six separate response
categories were used on both the 1990 and 2000 Census
questionnaires for Asians: Asian Indian, Chinese, Filipino, Japanese, Korean, and Vietnamese. For the 2000
Census, a separate "other Asian" response category
was used, with a write-in area in which respondents
could indicate a specific Asian group or subgroup not
included on the questionnaire. Using this reporting
structure, the 2000 Census showed that, of the 281.4
million people counted, 11.9 million (4.2%) reported
themselves as being Asian (U.S. Bureau of the Census,
2000). This number included 10.2 million (3.6%) who
were designated as Asian alone and 1.7 million (0.6%)
who reported Asian in addition to one or more other
races. Of significance, however, is that the Census
showed that the Asian population increased faster than
the total population between 1990 and 2000 (Barnes &
Bennett, 2002)—a 48% to 72% increase for the Asian
population, depending on whether the Asian alone or in
combination categories were used, versus a 13% increase in the total population. In addition to being fast
growing, a profile of the Asian population in the United
States (U.S. Bureau of the Census, 2001) showed that
they are relatively well educated (44% had a bachelor's

Requests for reprints should be sent to Tony M. Wong, Unity
Health System, Department of Physical Medicine and Rehabilitation, 89 Genesee St., Rochester, NY 14611. E-mail: twong@
unityhealth.org

degree or higher, 86% had at least a high school diploma) and economically viable (record low poverty rate of 10.7% in 1999; 53% households owned their homes).

Despite the trends and categorization schemes mentioned, the use of the term *Asian* or *Asian American* can be quite misleading, as it might obfuscate the fact that this can be a very diverse and heterogeneous group. For example, although the six specific Asian groups used on the U.S. Census questionnaire do encompass nearly 90% of the classification of Asian and Pacific Islander from the 1990 Census (Hing, 1993), there are actually 32 distinct cultural groups underlying this rubric. Although there are similarities in racial features and cultural values among the various Asian American groups, there are also discrete differences that need to be understood. The cultural diversity of Asian Americans (both between and within group) presents a significant challenge to the clinical neuropsychologist who is evaluating an individual from that group. Because there is little literature and research with respect to the neuropsychological assessment of Asian Americans, the clinician unfamiliar with this group would be hard pressed to organize a set of appropriate procedures with appropriate norms to perform a comprehensive assessment (Wong, 2000). The risk, then, would be that the neuropsychologist would either be unable to engage and assess the patient or perform a less than adequate assessment that may well be based on inappropriate assumptions with respect to the individual's background and test performances.

The goal of this article, then, is to provide clinical neuropsychologists who might be unfamiliar with Asian American peoples and cultures with some basic knowledge and principles by which to guide their work with people from these groups. This is done by (a) familiarizing the reader with information and a description of specific Asian subgroups, (b) providing a context within which neuropsychological test selection and interpretation can be determined, and (c) providing practical suggestions for working with Asian American clients in a neuropsychological setting. It should be noted that, for the purposes of this article, only four of the largest Asian subgroups (Chinese, Filipino, Japanese, and Korean) and one of the most rapidly growing subgroups, the Vietnamese and other Southeast Asians, is discussed in any detail. Perhaps as an illustration of the fundamental heterogeneity of what is termed *Asian* is the fact that not all agree with the inclusion criteria for who would be included under this grouping. Hing (1993), for example, noted that, because of geographic distance from the rest of Asia, their unique racial fea-

tures, and their distinctive cultures, some researchers do not consider Asian Indians and Filipinos as being appropriately grouped with the other Asian subgroups. However, for this article, the choice was made to focus on those whose heritage is from the more eastern geographic regions of Asia. Therefore, this should not be interpreted as a statement on the legitimacy of Indians as a significant Asian culture.

Asian Americans: Similarities and Differences

Although both intergroup and intragroup differences among the various Asian American subgroups are often ignored, some general common characteristics need to be understood, especially by professionals who are from a more Western cultural mindset. In contrast to modern Western culture, in which the individual is the most fundamental and important unit, traditional Asian cultures place greater emphasis on the family or extended family as the primary organism (Wong, 2000). Thus, in traditional Asian families, the family unit, which is likely to be extended, is more highly valued than the individual (Lee, 1996). The emotions or wishes of the individual are to be moderated and controlled, and conformity and mutual dependence are treasured. Moreover, the family system is hierarchical, with filial piety, respect for the elderly, and respect for authority being of great importance (Wong, 2000). However, as del Carmen (1990) aptly noted, there has been a gradual shift away from an extended family structure and toward the nuclear family in contemporary Asia. Therefore, the traditional Asian emphasis on the extended family and on group versus individual orientation might be in flux. Nevertheless, knowing some of these cultural tendencies may help the neuropsychologist to understand certain behaviors, particularly behaviors that might appear nonnormative from a Western perspective. For example, Wong noted that the oldest son of an elderly Asian woman, who has pronounced behavioral and cognitive deficits secondary to an aggressive lobar dementia, might decline the recommendation of the neuropsychologist to place her in a long-term care facility and instead decide to take her home with him, despite the fact that he has a family with three young children.

Although the various Asian American peoples may share certain common cultural characteristics and even physical appearance similarities, it would be a serious mistake to view them as a homogenous group. Unfortunately, intraethnic differences among the Asian American groups have received little attention (Lee, 1996; Uba, 1994), and, until recently, most of the research in psychology and mental health has focused on Chinese Americans and Japanese Americans. Nevertheless, neuropsychologists and others who work with Asian American clients would be well advised to be aware of significant between-group differences as well as within-group differences with factors such as acculturation, language or English proficiency, migration history, educational attainment, and other factors. This is crucial information not only for the purpose of facilitating an atmosphere of understanding and rapport, but also for providing the appropriate context or baseline by which to determine an appropriate assessment and eventual interpretation of such. It is for this purpose that the following sections are offered. They describe some of the larger Asian American groups whose origins are from the Eastern regions of Asia. These descriptions are not intended as exhaustive or comprehensive summaries of these cultural groups, but rather as a starting point of knowledge or understanding for those who may not be familiar with the various Asian American groups.

Chinese Americans

The Chinese are the largest Asian subgroup in America, making up 23.7% of the total Asian population in the United States (U.S. Bureau of the Census, 2000). Substantial growth was seen in this group in the decade from 1990 to 2000, as its population in this country increased by 43.8% to 2,432,585. This group is also likely to be the Asian subgroup that has been present in America the longest, with reports of the presence of Chinese on the continent not long after the arrival of Europeans.

The first period of large-scale immigration of Chinese into this country occurred after the discovery of gold in California in 1848, along with the need for manual labor for railroad construction. Large numbers of Chinese men, particularly from the southern coastal province of Guangdong, immigrated to the western United States (Chan, 1991). However, their growing presence and competition with White laborers resulted in anti-Chinese sentiment and the enactment of exclusion laws, including the Chinese Exclusion Act of 1882. These laws prevented Chinese laborers from bringing over their wives and families, severely limited their rights (e.g., citizenship, land ownership), and had the net effect of halting the flow of Chinese immigration (from a high of 107,488 Chinese residents in 1880

to 61,639 in 1920; Gaw, 1993). From 1930 to 1965, because of a series of changes in immigration laws and policies, more Chinese women were allowed to enter America, leading to reunification and establishment of families of Chinese heritage in the United States. After 1965, the pattern of Chinese immigration into the United States shifted. Many came over as families. Especially in more recent years, ethnic Chinese from more diverse areas of the world have been immigrating. These diverse areas included not only China, Hong Kong, and Taiwan, but also areas of Southeast Asia (e.g., Vietnam, Laos, and Cambodia). In addition, a number of so-called overseas Chinese from such countries as Japan, Korea, Philippines, Singapore, Malaysia, as well as countries in South America and Europe, joined the rapid influx of Chinese immigrants (Lee, 1996). The sociological makeup of Chinese Americans has been influenced significantly by immigration policies and patterns (Wong, 2000), resulting in marked heterogeneity with respect to English proficiency, immigration status, social norms, and other such factors related to acculturation. For example, those who descended from the early immigrants of the 19th century largely had their origins from the rural villages outside of Guangzhou in Guangdong province and were primarily speakers of Cantonese or Taishanese. The more elderly among these—many of whom still live in the various Chinatowns in our country—have little formal education and retain many of their native cultural traditions. However, despite their relatively lengthy tenure as residents in the United States, they may be very poor English speakers. In contrast, more recent Chinese immigrants are more diverse socioeconomically and educationally and may speak Mandarin, the national language of China, and may have some basic proficiency in English, particularly if they are well educated. Country of origin is also an important factor. Among the more recent immigrants, for example, those from Singapore may be more likely to adapt to American culture compared with those from China because of Singapore's more Westernized culture relative to China (Lee, 1996). neuropsychologists, then, need to take great care in assessing the acculturation and language proficiency of a Chinese American client in preparation of a valid neuropsychological assessment because of the heterogeneity of this group.

Despite the diversity of the Chinese American population in the United States, there are certain common cultural characteristics, especially among those who are less acculturated, that are useful for neuropsychologists to understand when working with clients of Chinese descent. The historical sociocultural influence of the literate traditions of Confucianism, Taoism, and Buddhism on Chinese society is one of these elements. For example, a Confucian worldview, with its emphasis on family harmony and social relationships with relatively well-defined roles, underlies a strong loyalty to the family and the group. In a hierarchical scheme, explicit rules govern key relationships: The individual is subordinate to the group, the young to the aged, the living to the ancestors, the wife to the husband, the children to the parents, and the daughter-in-law to the mother-in-law (Jung, 1998). Because of this emphasis on the family or group, mental illness (or any behaviors suggesting mental disorder) is very stigmatizing and viewed as a shameful reflection on family. Thus, there is a strong tendency within this culture to minimize or hide mental health-related problems, with a preference toward handling the issues within the family without help from outsiders. Elliot, Di Minno, Lam, and Tu (1996) noted, for example, that the Chinese respond to memory and associated problems in the elderly by either viewing these as normal consequences of growing old or, alternatively, interpreting the signs and symptoms of dementia as indicative of a mental disorder.

These cultural characteristics may explain some stereotypical behaviors of a Chinese client in a psychological or neuropsychological context and how some of those behaviors can be addressed. Respect for authority and for those who are older may be manifested in a reluctance to speak directly about another, especially to express disagreement, disapproval, or concern. The patient or his or her family members may not volunteer critical information regarding behavioral or even cognitive symptoms because of a fear of stigmatization unless the neuropsychologist sensitively probes and initiates the discussion. The neuropsychologist is likely to be viewed as the "expert doctor," whose recommendations or preferences will be taken very seriously by the patient or his or her family. It behooves the neuropsychologist, then, to be aware of his or her own stimulus value to them (Wong, 2000). Conversely, despite the recommendations of the respected professional, families of Chinese patients may decide to take them home for long-term care at great inconvenience and disruption to their personal lives rather than to place them in a facility because of strong cultural obligations to care for one's elders. The prevalence of somatization symptoms among Chinese has been reported by a number of investigators (Gaw, 1993), ostensibly because of the explanation that physical complaints are more socially acceptable to Chinese than an expression of emotional complaints. Neuropsychologists can take advantage of this cultural preference for physical manifestations and

explanations of behavior by framing neurobehavioral sequelae of brain injury or neurologic disease as symptoms of a medical problem rather than as mental health problems. Chinese patients or their families will often turn to traditional Chinese remedies or medicines if they believe that Western-style medicine has not been effective. This is rooted in centuries of classic and folk Chinese medicine. Wong suggested that sometimes the physician can attempt a compromise by offering to allow the patient to take the Chinese remedy as long as an evaluation ensures it does not have any adverse effects or is contraindicated by Western medicine. This way, instead of creating an unnecessarily antagonistic situation, a cultural preference that is not harmful can be facilitated and can foster an atmosphere of respect and greater rapport between the practitioner and patient.

Filipino Americans

The Filipinos are the second largest Asian group in the United States. According to the 2000 U.S. Census, there are approximately 1,850,000 Filipino Americans—a 31.5% increase from 1990 (U.S. Bureau of the Census, 2000). According to Araneta (1996), the states with the highest concentration of Filipino Americans are California (52%), Hawaii (12%), Illinois (4.6%), New York (4.4.%), New Jersey (3.8%), and Washington (3.1%).

Filipinos are a heterogeneous culture with a population spread over 7,000 islands. There are 75 dialects and 8 major languages, the 4 most prominent being Tagalog, Ilocano, Visayan, and English (Ponce & Forman, 1980). Filipino culture is rich with strong influences from Malaysia, Spain, and, more recently, America. The Malay influence on Filipinos is manifest in their belief in fatalism, or *bahala na*, magic, clannishness, and the emphasis on the extended family (Ponce & Forman, 1980). The Spanish influence is seen in Catholicism, hierarchical relationships, and a strong deference to authority (Ponce & Forman, 1980). The adoption of English as a major language and the emulation of Western fashions are influences from America (Ponce & Forman, 1980).

The three major subcultural groups in the Philippines are the Tagalogs, the Ilocanos, and the Visayans. These subcultures are grouped by the language they speak and the location where they live. The Tagalogs have the strongest Spanish influence and tend to be the highest educated, most urban, and most Westernized. Ilocanos are primarily farmers who are described as being hardworking. The Visayans are known to be festive, sensual, and colorful (Ponce & Forsman, 1980).

The vast majority of Filipinos are multilingual, speaking their native dialect, Tagalog (the national language), and English. The mandatory primary and secondary educational system in the Philippines goes to the 10th grade. Approximately 29% of high school graduates continue on to college (International Bureau of Education, 2001X). English is the primary language spoken in schools from the fourth grade. Thus, unlike other Asian cultures, Filipinos tend to have the strongest English listening comprehension and speaking skills. Actual skill level, however, varies depending on the level and quality of education received. Despite mandatory exposure to English, most Filipinos are most comfortable speaking their own dialect, and comprehension is generally superior to expressive skills.

There have been three waves of Filipino immigration to the United States. The first wave of immigrants, who arrived from 1906–1934, were laborers who came to work the plantations of Hawaii, the orchards of California, and the fisheries of the northeastern states (Araneta, 1996). The second wave of Filipino immigration occurred from 1945–1965 after Congress granted citizenship to Filipinos who fought for the United States military in World War II. This wave of immigrants consisted of servicemen and their brides and students and professionals attracted by the growing U.S. economy (Araneta, 1996). The third and current wave of immigration began in 1965 after passage of the Immigration and Nationality Act Amendments of 1965 amended the early restrictions on Asian immigrants, and this wave is still going strong. From 1978–1998, an estimated 1.3 million Filipinos immigrated to the United States, which makes up 20% of all Asian immigration during this time (Le, 2001). This wave of immigration, known as the "brain drain," consisted of many middle-class, well-educated Filipinos who were critical of Marcos's corrupt government and who could not find decent jobs in the Philippines, despite having college degrees. Thus, they sought better opportunities in the United States (Takaki, 1995). Other primary motivators for immigration were the poor economic conditions of the Philippines and family reunification, because the extended family is the nuclear family in Filipino culture (Ponce & Forman, 1980).

Similar to the experience of most immigrants, integrating into American society has not been easy for many Filipino Americans. There is a high degree of underemployment; many with professional degrees from the Philippines faced discrimination on their arrival, and others could not meet strict licensure requirements

or pass rigorous board examinations (Takaki, 1995). There appears to be a bimodal distribution in educational status, with both a high percentage of Filipino Americans having some college education (47%–53%) as well as relatively high percentages who have not completed high school (28% foreign born, 32% American born; Alegado, 1987). Although similar to other Asian groups in which the median household income is higher than Whites, this figure is deceiving. Filipino American families are generally larger, with 33% having more than five members, and there are more persons per household in the workforce. In addition, among Asians, Filipino Americans have a higher representation in lower income categories (Araneta, 1996).

According to Marsella, Escudero, and Gordon (1971), some assimilation difficulties of Filipino Americans can be attributed to cultural beliefs—such as *bahala na* or thinking that one has little control over one's destiny, which is simply in the fate of God—because such beliefs are opposed to American values of future orientation, drive for excellence, and economic development through determined effort. Still, a growing number of Filipino Americans hold professional jobs. Nursing is one such occupation toward which many have gravitated. Others have capitalized on the increased need for geriatric care by operating family care home businesses.

In terms of beliefs toward psychiatric disorders, traditional Filipino culture attaches much stigma to disorders of mental illness that are generally perceived to result from weakness of the will or frailty of character (Santa Rita, 1993). Other common beliefs are that only the dangerously insane require psychiatric treatment or that mental illness is caused by "bad blood" or familial discord (Santa Rita, 1993).

Thus, when working with Filipino Americans, it is important that the clinician thoroughly explain the purpose of the meeting while using a problem-solving approach (Ponce & Forman, 1980). It is also recommended that the clinician take on the role of the expert who gives direct advice, at least initially, because this style of interaction is compatible with the cultural tendency of deferring to authority (Ponce & Forman, 1980). Other cultural values that may be salient in the context of providing mental health services to Filipino Americans include *pakikisama,* or avoidance of giving offense or openly disagreeing (Ponce & Forman, 1980). This value, in tandem with a deference to authority, will often manifest itself in the Filipino American client nodding his or her head in agreement with the clinician but not following through with advice, because it would be impolite to disagree with an authority figure. Probing and allowing choices may be useful to learn the true desires of the Filipino American client. *Amor propio*, or fragile sense of self-worth, renders the Filipino American client vulnerable to negative remarks; thus, communicating praise, acceptance, and support is crucial for successful therapeutic interactions (Ponce & Forman, 1980).

Vietnamese Americans and Other Southeast Asian Americans

The fastest growing Asian group in the United States is the Vietnamese. They numbered 1,122,528 in the 2000 U.S. Census, showing an 82.7% increase in their population from 1990 to 2000 and moving from the fifth largest Asian group in the United States to the third largest. They also represent the most geographically concentrated among the Asian groups because of the relatively brief timeline of Vietnamese immigration, with sizable communities in California and Texas. The Vietnamese are often grouped with other Southeast Asian peoples such as Cambodians (Khmer), Laotians, and Hmong because of the geographic proximity of their native lands and their similar migration history. Between one third and one half of Vietnamese Americans are of Chinese ancestry (Gondo, 2003).

A substantial portion of the Vietnamese American population immigrated to the United States as refugees from South Vietnam after the fall of Saigon in 1975. This first wave of immigration, from 1975–1977, also included other Southeast Asians, particularly Cambodians and Highland Laotians (Hmong). The second major wave of Southeast Asian immigration occurred from 1978–1980, as the region continued to be plagued by war and economic hardship (D'Avanzo, 1997), including the overthrow of the Khmer Rouge regime by the Vietnamese. Because of this history, the Vietnamese have the highest ratio of recent immigrants among the five major Asian American groups (Gondo, 2003), with 33% having immigrated within the past 10 years. Despite this high ratio of recent immigration and concomitant high rate of households living below the poverty level, there is noticeable variability in the educational and socioeconomic background within this group. Some, particularly those who came over with the first wave, were highly educated, Western-trained Vietnamese professionals who adjusted fairly well to America and have been successful academically here (Kinzie & Leung, 1993). Other Southeast Asian refugees were from a rural background with little formal education, and they have had a more difficult time adjusting.

Unfortunately, because Vietnamese and other peoples who have geographic origins from the same general area are often grouped and described together as "Southeast Asians" or "Indochinese," the ethnic and cultural diversity of this group is often not well understood. Neuropsychologists who work with people from this background are encouraged to educate themselves regarding the specific relevant subgroup. For example, Vietnamese culture and history have had long and significant influence from China (Leung & Boehnlein, 1996). Thus, as in Chinese culture, the spiritual life of Vietnamese people has been shaped by Confucianism, Buddhism, and Taoism (Do, 1999). In contrast, the religion and language of Cambodia and Laos have been influenced by India (Kinzie & Leung, 1993). Thus, elements of Hindu Brahmanism, as well as Buddhism, are part of the religious culture of these countries.

As with other Asian cultures, Southeast Asian social structure is based on the extended family, with social order highly stratified and hierarchical. McKenzie-Pollock (1996) noted that this is even reflected in language, as, for example, a different word for eating is used in the Khmer language depending on the rank of the person being referred to. For the Vietnamese, *Hieu*, or filial piety, is one of the basic virtues and refers to the notion of love, care, and respect that children give to their parents (Do, 1999). This emphasis on and value of familial relationships is reflected in the strong preference toward addressing problems, especially those of a psychological nature, within the family. Related to this is the stigmatization of mental illness (or related entities), as this is a potential source of shame to the Southeast Asian family with possible social repercussions, including ostracism and the inability to find suitable marital partners for family members (Kinzie & Leung, 1993). Moreover, the concept of psychotherapy or seeing a psychologist of any type is unfamiliar to most Southeast Asians. Nishio and Bilmes (1998) wrote that, when Southeast Asian refugees come to a traditional mental health agency, they perceive the referral as a choice initiated by physicians, social service workers, the court, or other public health personnel and not their own choice; they will seek mental health help on their own only as a last resort. Neuropsychologists working with Southeast Asian patients are well advised, then, to engage the family as well as the patient and to gain their trust.

Southeast Asians also have been known, as with other Asian groups, to be prone toward somatization. For example, Lao, Mien, and Hmong refugee populations have been observed to present to health care settings with a high prevalence of somatic or bodily complaints, yet with no eventual findings of physical cause for such complaints (Moore, Keopraseuth, Leung, & Chao, 1997). Some of this is ostensibly because of the culturally based belief, common to the Southeast Asian peoples, that the health of the body and mind are inseparable. Related to this is the notion that mental illness has a metaphysical cause, with the spirit world and supernatural forces such as "bad wind" affecting physical and mental health (Nishio & Bilmes, 1998). Many have noted that, because of this tendency toward somatization and because of the high proportion of Southeast Asians who have been exposed to war trauma, mental health professionals should be careful to assess for posttraumatic stress disorder and depression (e.g., Boehnlein, Leung, & Kinzie, 1997; Leung, Boehnlein, & Kinzie, 1997; Moore et al., 1997).

In working with Vietnamese Americans, knowledge of communication patterns is important. Like many Asian groups, Vietnamese Americans are respectful of persons in high positions, such as doctors. They are also nonconfrontational. When speaking to a Vietnamese American, a neuropsychologist should be aware that, in the Vietnamese language, *da*, or yes, means not only that one is in agreement, but also that simply "I am politely listening to you" (Nguyen & Kehmeier, 1980). Another common response by Vietnamese Americans to authority figures is a silent smile. This can indicate that the client either does not agree or does not understand; however, out of politeness, the client will not contradict the speaker or ask for clarification (Nguyen & Kehmeier, 1980). Given this dual meaning of yes and the ambiguity of a silent smile, clinicians need to be cautious in interpreting responses of the Vietnamese Americans, and questions may need further probing.

Korean Americans

Korean Americans are the fourth largest Asian group in the United States. According to the 2000 U.S. Census, there are approximately 1,077,000 Korean Americans, which is a 34.8% increase from 1990 (U.S. Bureau of the Census, 1990, 2000). Among all American ethnic groups, not just Asians, Koreans Americans have the distinction of being the most highly educated and having the highest median income (Gondo, 2003).

As with many Asian groups, Korean immigration can be divided into three periods. The first wave of immigrants consisted of poor male farmers from what is now known as North Korea. They came as contract laborers to Hawaii plantations with the intention of accumulating wealth and returning to Korea (B. L. C. Kim,

1993). From 1910–1924, the immigration of picture brides from Southern Korea—women whose marriages to the initial wave of immigrants were arranged by families and characterized by an exchange of pictures—followed. The first wave of immigration ended with the Oriental Exclusion Act of 1924, which prevented further immigration from Asia (B. L. C. Kim, 1993). The second wave of immigration occurred from 1950–1965, after the Korean War. This wave consisted primarily of war orphans and Amerasian children adopted by American parents, as well as Korean women who married U.S. servicemen. A number of students and physicians also immigrated during this period (L. I. C. Kim, 1996). The third wave of Korean immigration, consisting primarily of nuclear families from South Korea, began in 1965 with the Immigration and Naturalization Act Amendments and continues to the present. There is also a wider range of socioeconomic and educational levels among this last wave, with 50% holding professional, technical, or managerial positions in Korea (L. I. C. Kim, 1996). From 1971–1998, 738,035 persons emigrated from South Korea, constituting 11% of all Asian immigrants during this period (Gondo, 2003). In 1990, 72% of all Korean Americans were foreign born (U.S. Bureau of the Census, 2000).

The primary motivation for the third wave of Korean immigration is the lack of professional positions. Koreans are among the best educated of Asian groups, with 88% of children in preprimary education and 68% continuing past secondary to tertiary education (International Bureau of Education, 2001b). Academics in Korea is highly competitive, which reflects Confucian beliefs that place a high value on education (Gondo, 2003). Despite an educated population, Korean cities were overcrowded, with more qualified workers in professional and managerial positions than available. Thus, many sought better opportunities in the United States. Unfortunately, only approximately one third could find comparable jobs in the United States (L. I. C. Kim, 1996). A significant factor is the language barrier; 90% of Korean immigrants speak only Korean and thus had to learn English on their arrival. Most Koreans, however, can read and write English, which is required in their academic curriculum (Harvey & Chung, 1980). Discrimination and strict professional licensure requirements are also important factors in Korean American underemployment.

Many Korean Americans have dealt with this adversity through self-employment. A relatively high percentage own and run grocery stores, liquor marts, laundries, gas stations, and souvenir shops (Takaki, 1995). These businesses were financed primarily from money that Korean Americans brought with them, although others financed their businesses with money from Korean cooperative credit associations or bank loans (Takaki, 1995). Such businesses require long hours and are often located in unsavory parts of the city. However, the mentality of the first generation is to work hard so that the children can attend good colleges and become professionals like the parents were in Korea. Korean immigration has been slowing recently because of the strong South Korean economy.

As with other Asian cultures, Koreans place a strong emphasis on family and the group, the latter resulting from the value of *in'gan,* or a connectedness with others (Harvey & Chung, 1980). They are a proud people who are highly sensitive to the opinions of others, thus *che-myun,* or "face saving," is important to them (Harvey & Chung, 1980). At the core of Korean culture are what appear to be contradictory beliefs. As mentioned previously, their emphasis on education, work ethic, and strong drive to succeed are rooted in Confucian beliefs. Role gratification is important, and Koreans experience much guilt if they feel they have failed to live up to their expectations (Harvey & Chung, 1980). Conversely, Koreans are also fatalists, believing in *p'alcha,* that a person's role and life status is predetermined (L. I. C. Kim, 1996), and *chaesu,* or destiny (Harvey & Chung, 1980). According to Harvey and Chung, the fatalistic belief of Koreans helps them to deal with failures with hope for change.

Many Koreans believe that mental illness results from family disharmony. Thus, the mentally ill are treated within the family by reducing demands and responsibilities. Koreans may seek outside treatment only if the person's behavior becomes unmanageable or aggressive (Harvey & Chung, 1980). Other Koreans, particularly from more rural areas, believe that mental illness is caused by evil or vengeful spirits or imbalances of *yin* and *yang* within the body. These people tend to seek treatment from shamans or traditional Chinese medicine (L. I. C. Kim, 1996). When working with Korean Americans, L. I. C. Kim recommended that clinicians be directive, be accepting of the person's belief system, and counter shame by reframing help-seeking behavior as an effort to maintain the family's good name.

Japanese Americans

The Japanese are the fifth largest Asian group in the United States and account for 7.8% of all Asians in the United States. According to the 2000 U.S. Census,

there are approximately 800,000 Japanese Americans. Unlike other Asian groups, the Japanese population in America has declined in comparison with the 1990 Census by approximately 6% (U.S. Bureau of the Census, 2000). This decline has been attributed to small family sizes and low immigration rates (Ellington, 2001).

The majority of Japanese Americans can trace their heritage to immigration from the turn of the century. The initial wave of immigrants—the *dekasegi,* or sojourners—were poor male farmers with limited education who arrived from 1885–1907 (Kitano, 1995). Burdened with an increased tax load from the Meiji emperor, they sought to accrue wealth in America, where higher wages were paid for contract plantation laborers, and eventually to return to Japan. These immigrants settled in Hawaii and the west coast states of California, Oregon, and Washington (Matsui, 1993). However, as with most get-rich-quick schemes, wealth was not to be attained, and the majority did not return.

The second wave of immigrants, arriving from 1907–1924, was composed of laborers who planned for permanent residency. These immigrants made a quick transition from laborers to business owners (J. S. Fujii, Fukushima, & Yamamoto, 1996). After both waves of immigrants were "picture brides," women who immigrated for arranged marriages. The majority of immigration from Japan came to a halt in 1924, when the Oriental Exclusion Act was passed.

Since 1924, relatively few Japanese have immigrated to America, even after the passage of the Immigration and Nationality Act Amendments of 1965 amended the early restrictions on Asian immigrants. Anti-Japanese sentiment after World War II and Japan's booming economy in latter part of 20th century are the primary reasons for the reduced immigration. Immigrants during this time have generally been military brides, adventurous souls who experienced American life as students, and expatriate executives (Gondo, 2003). In addition, since the economic boom, there have been a relatively large number of executives of U.S. subsidiaries of Japanese companies who do 3- to 5-year tours of duties but still maintain Japanese citizenship. These people number approximately 100,000 (Gondo, 2003).

Given that approximately 78% of Japanese Americans are native born, they are among the most acculturated of the Asian groups (Kitano, 1995). Most young to middle-aged adults are third (*sansei*), fourth (*yonsei*), and fifth (*gosei*) generation, whereas a large number of young and middle-aged elderly are second generation (*nisei*). A subset of this latter group, the *kibei,* were born in the United States, but were sent back to Japan for their education. Another implication of the Japanese immigration pattern to the United States is that, with the exception of few *issei* (first generation), *kibei,* and more recent immigrants, English is the primary language.

The English speaking abilities of the more recent immigrants, however, can be highly variable. The educational system in Japan is one of the best and most competitive in the world and is particularly strong in math. The literacy rate is roughly 95%. (In the United States, it is 88%.) A Japanese high school degree has been estimated to be equivalent to 2 years of American college (Ellington, 2001). The Japanese learn to read and write English, but speaking English is generally not part of the regular curriculum. Those who study and work abroad must have at least a minimum competency for listening comprehension, although speaking is usually less developed. Among the least educated and proficient in English are likely to be military brides.

The Japanese have assimilated well in America because of their values of hard work and thrift and a strong emphasis on education, which are very similar to the Western Protestant ethic (Rogers & Izutsu, 1980). In the United States, the Japanese American mean and median household income is estimated to be 20%–25% higher than other Asian Pacific Islander groups, which as a whole is slightly higher than Whites. Only 3.4% live below the poverty line (U.S. Bureau of the Census, 1990, 2000).

Culturally, Japanese place a strong allegiance to family and the group. At the heart of traditional Japanese culture are the complementary values of *amae,* which is a dependency and presumption of another's benevolence (Doi, 1962), and *on,* a sense of obligation (Lebra, 1969). *Amae,* or "sweet," characterizes the dependency of the infant on the mother. This assumption also can be applied to the group to which one belongs. *On* fosters interdependence among peers, whereas in vertical relationships, the person in authority assumes the responsibility of looking out for his or her subordinates. Once established, *on* is reversible only by treacherous behavior; thus, the Japanese tend to be interpersonally guarded, because including someone in one's personal circle holds strong obligations (Rogers & Izutsu, 1980).

Much of stereotypically Japanese behavior can be tied to the strong allegiance to the group. Indirect speaking, often interpreted as evasiveness, is associated with a concern for other's opinions. Japanese do not want to offend and avoid outward disagreement; thus, they throw out feelers to elicit opinions. In this regard,

attending to nonverbals, often emitted in Zenlike silence, is a crucial aspect of communication. Clannishness results from a strong allegiance to the group and guardedness toward outsiders. Similarly, the external locus of the Japanese also is related to the motivation of shame. There is a strong drive to bring honor to the family and group. Conversely, behaviors or characteristics shunned by society, including mental illness, are often hidden so as not to bring shame on the family (Rogers & Izutsu, 1980). Cultural implications for neuropsychologists are that Japanese Americans are less likely to seek services for mental illness because of shame (J. S. Fujii et al., 1996). This reticence does not mean that Japanese Americans have less psychopathology than other ethnic groups (Kuo, 1984). Instead, they have an inordinately high tolerance for unusual behaviors demonstrated by mentally ill family members and will care for them from within the family system. External resources may be contacted only if behaviors become highly disruptive (J. S. Fujii et al., 1996). Japanese Americans often present with concerns of physical illness or academic and vocational concerns that are more acceptable (J. S. Fujii et al., 1996; Tracey, leong, & Glidden, 1986). Thus, when Japanese Americans seek treatment, they may be at a higher severity level or may be experiencing more stress than they may be presenting (Rogers & Izutsu, 1980). Assuring confidentiality is important to assuage issues of shame.

Practical Guidelines

The following are practical guidelines for neuropsychological testing with Asian American people. Steps to neuropsychological testing include (a) cultural education and preparation, (b) determination of whether cultural factors are relevant, (c) information gathering, (d) test selection and test administration, (e) test interpretation, and (f) report writing.

The first step in working with Asian Americans is to be adequately prepared. Preparation includes being aware of American Psychological Association (APA) ethical and cultural guidelines in working with minority cultures (APA, 1993, 2002), as well as other criteria for multicultural competency (Hansen, Pepitone-Arreola-Rockwell, & Greene, 2000); being knowledgeable in behavioral neurology and neuropsychiatry; and, most important, having an adequate knowledge base about the client's cultural background. The latter can be obtained by reading cultural anthropology books, speaking to colleagues or clients of a given culture, and attending cultural seminars (Wong, 2000). Knowledge about cultural beliefs, traditions, values, behavioral presentation, and life experiences will be useful in developing a rapport and will place the client and his or her family at ease. Knowledge about the country's educational system, immigration patterns, employment and socioeconomic status, and gender roles is important for developing a context within which to interpret test scores. Both are important when conceptualizing implications of findings for the client and family and making culturally sensitive and relative recommendations. For example, knowing that most Asian American cultures have a high tolerance for disruptive behaviors from family members because of shame and stigma and that they generally seek professional assistance only when the family member becomes a danger or unbearable would alert the clinician that any person brought in by the family is likely to be at a relatively high level of psychopathology. In addition, stress levels may not mirror the emotional presentation of the family, particularly for the less expressive Japanese Americans.

The second step is determining to what extent cultural factors are relevant for each client. Two important factors are English proficiency and acculturation, which, although separate, are generally highly correlated (Wong et al., 2000). These factors would be very salient for the overwhelming majority of immigrants and less of a factor with each subsequent generation living in the United States.

The extent to which these factors are salient in a client will determine two important decisions for the clinician: (a) Should the client be referred elsewhere?, and (b) Is an interpreter needed? The decision to refer elsewhere depends on the clinician's comfort level, knowledge base, competency, and expertise in working with persons of a certain culture, as well as the availability of a better alternative. Certainly, if the clinician is working with a Korean American who speaks little English and knows of a Korean speaking, Korean American neuropsychologist, it behooves the clinician to refer. When determining the need for an interpreter, a general heuristic is to seek an interpreter if the client is not comfortable in either English comprehension or expression. If the clinician would like to determine English comprehension, quick screens include administering the Auditory Comprehension subtest of the Boston Diagnostic Aphasia Examination (Goodglass & Kaplan, 1987) or sampling items on the Peabody Picture Vocabulary Test–Revised (Dunn & Dunn, 1981)—the latter to estimate an age-level score.

Even if the client reports being comfortable with English, the clinician should consider an interpreter for interviewing family members who may not speak English fluently. An interpreter whose ethnic background is the same as the client also may be useful in helping the clinician determine what is normal behavior for that culture. Issues with translators are reviewed elsewhere (Sandoval & Duran, 1998; Wong et al., 2000).

Given the problems with testing persons of different cultures, particularly immigrants and persons for whom English is a second language, obtaining accurate and thorough background information is essential to understanding potential neuropsychological sequelae of neurological disorders (Artiola I Fortuny, 2003). Thus, thorough knowledge about cognitive, behavioral, emotional, and psychiatric sequelae associated with specific lesion locations and neurological disorders are useful for guiding information gathering. When working with Asian Americans, neuropsychologists may need to be more directive than usual, as many of these clients may be less likely or able to spontaneously provide pertinent information to the clinician. In this regard, gathering information from collaterals is very important, particularly in determining what changes in behavior, if any, occurred after a neurological event and what behaviors are considered normal for that culture. Again, given the questionable validity of American-developed tests on less acculturated or non-English speaking clients, detailed collateral accounts may be the best information for conceptualizing the presence or severity of cognitive deficits (D. Fujii, Umetsu, Schwartz, & Hostetter, 2002).

Two other issues with cultural implications are assessing for premorbid abilities and depression. Estimating premorbid abilities can be challenging because conventional methods of estimation, such as reading tests or current occupation, may not be valid for immigrant populations. Information that would be useful in estimating premorbid abilities includes (a) where in the native country a person was born and raised; (b) date and reason for immigrating to America; (c) occupation and educational level in the native country; (d) academic achievement in the native country; (e) parent's occupation and educational level in the native country; (f) occupation and education in America; (g) occupation and education of siblings or children in America; and (h) comparison of client's intelligence to family members—for example, more difficulty in school than siblings. In terms of depression, which can affect attention, concentration, and memory (for a review, see Lezak, 1995), clinicians should be knowledgeable about a particular culture's typical presentation of depression and common cultural reasons for being depressed.

Issues in test selection and administration, as well as interpretation, depend on the acculturation, English speaking ability, and education level of the client. Modifications to standard protocols often are necessary for immigrant populations with low levels of education who do not speak English well. However, within the context of a culturally sensitive interaction, the clinician can generally proceed in the usual manner for third generation Asian Americans, although some caution in interpretation should be maintained (Wong, 2000). More variability exists for second generation Asian Americans. The following guidelines are for working with the less acculturated who have poor English skills.

When selecting appropriate tests for less acculturated Asian Americans, the ideal is to administer tests developed and validated with a specific ethnic group, such as the Cognitive Assessment Screening Instrument (Teng et al., 1994) or Korean California Verbal Learning Test (J. K. Kim & Kang, 1999), or that have norms for that ethnic group, such as verbal fluency (Kempler, Teng, Dick, Taussig, & Davis, 1998). Tests of functional abilities, such as the Clinical Dementia Rating (Hughes, Berg, Danziger, Cohen, & Markan, 1982), that rate level of impairment on the basis of observations of different functional domains can minimize cultural bias. Unfortunately, very few of these tests are currently available. With an interpreter, test items such as the Rey Auditory Verbal Learning Test (Taylor, 1969) can be translated into the client's primary language. Although more fair, there are problems with interpretation because of a lack of normative data (for a review, see Fouad & Chan, 1999).

In this less than perfect world, the clinician will likely have to resort to using standard neuropsychological tests developed and normed only on American samples. There are several caveats when doing so. First, tests with obvious cultural biases should be avoided and substituted with less biased tests. For example, the Weshsler Adult Intelligence Scale–III (WAIS–III) Vocabulary subtest (Wechsler, 1997) is highly invalid for those with poor English comprehension or expression, whereas the Peabody Picture Vocabulary Test–Revised (Dunn & Dunn, 1981) and the Wechsler Adult Intelligence Scale–Revised (WAIS–R) as a Neuropsychological Instrument Vocabulary multiple choice subtest are better measures of receptive vocabulary in English (Kaplan, Fein, Morris, & Delis, 1991). Category fluency would result in less bias than the standard FAS (Controlled Oral Word Association Test) letter fluency test (Spreen & Benton, 1969). The clinician also should be aware of potential cultural biases for individual items. For example, many older Japanese, Korean, and Chinese persons can readily identify an abacus, the most difficult item on the Boston Naming Test (Kaplan,

Goodglass, & Weintraub, 1983). In terms of nonverbal tests, these are not as culturally fair as they may appear, particularly for those with education levels below the ninth grade (Artiola I Fortuny, 1997).

When testing Asian Americans who do not speak fluent English, nonstandardized approaches, whether in English or through an interpreter, may be necessary to ensure that the client understands the instructions. Nell (2000) argued for practitioners to start with the lowest item versus standard starting items on the WAIS–III when testing clients who are unfamiliar with Western tests to give them some practice with these unique tasks. Given the education level of many immigrant Asian Americans, Nell's recommendation may not be necessary, but it may be considered for those who are poorly educated. Another important aspect of test administration is observing for behaviors consistent with neurological syndromes.

A multimethod approach is recommended when interpreting neuropsychological test data (D. Fujii et al., 2002). Integrating data from different sources such as behavioral observations, history, medical reports, and collateral reports, in addition to neuropsychological test results, is the general approach of most clinicians. However, given the questionable validity and precision of neuropsychological test data for poorly acculturated and poor English speaking Asian Americans, the clinician must rely more heavily on consistency of overall presentation to neurobehavioral syndromes and on other sources of data for case conceptualization. Some questions to guide interpretation include (a) What functional deficits or behavioral changes does the family report after a neurological event?, (b) Did changes occur abruptly after a neurological event?, (c) Is the progression of deficits consistent with a known neurological disorder?, and (d) Are behavioral changes consistent with what is expected for a neurological event or diagnosis?

Although the ability of test results to estimate cognitive strengths and weaknesses in poorly acculturated Asian Americans is, at best, imprecise, we suggest some heuristics in test interpretation. First, if patients perform well on the selected American-developed and American-normed tests, some confidence can be placed in ruling out deficits. Second, if there are deficits, the clinician can be more confident of this rough estimate if the pattern is consistent with a known neurological syndrome or if the results are so discrepant that they cannot be explained entirely by cultural factors for that particular patient (Nell, 2000). Third, independent of test scores, learning potential, or the ability to improve performances on tests with experience, may be a good prognostic indicator of a person' ability to benefit from different training for rehabilitation (Nell, 2000). Tests that lend themselves to improvement over trials include Trail Making Test A and B (Army Individual Test Battery, 1944), WAIS–III Block Design and Digit Span (Wechsler, 1997), and the Wisconsin Card Sorting Test (Heaton, Chelune, & Talley, 1993).

When writing reports, it is important to stress the limitations of test interpretation and to amply qualify test results. In general, results are likely a low estimate of actual abilities, particularly for verbal tests if the client is not proficient in English. All nonstandardized test administrations should be documented. If test results are deemed to have poor validity, the clinician may need to emphasize functional abilities as described by collateral sources. Even if the Asian American client speaks fluent English and is highly acculturated, the clinician should be cautious in assuming that the predictive validity of test results is the same as for Whites. For example, studies have demonstrated that Chinese and Japanese Americans often attain higher occupational status than would be predicted by their level of intelligence (Flynn, 1991).

In general, but particularly for forensic cases, it is good practice to cite evidence for each conclusion made. Elucidating the thought processes is especially crucial when less weight is placed on neuropsychological test results because of cultural and language factors. In such cases, it may be useful to differentially qualify the confidence for each conclusion made. For example, the clinician may have different certainty levels about (a) whether the client's presentation is consistent with a neurological disorder, (b) the nature and severity of cognitive deficits, (c) the client's functional abilities to return to work or live independently, (d) the client's ability to make informed decisions, or (e) the client's understanding and appreciation of court proceedings. In making recommendations, the client's cultural context always should be considered.

Summary and Conclusion

Asian Americans, although sharing many cultural and physical similarities, are a diverse and heterogeneous group that defies simple characterization. As the population of this group in the United States continues to grow, neuropsychologists are more likely to be placed in a situation in which they are asked to conduct an evaluation of an Asian American client or patient. Without appropriate background information, knowledge, and understanding of the cultural context from

which a particular patient comes, the validity of the neuropsychological evaluation may be at risk. This article provides merely a starting point for neuropsychologists who are unfamiliar with how to approach an evaluation with a client or patient of Asian descent. As such, only a cursory and general overview of the characteristics of the major Asian American subgroups, major issues relevant to the neuropsychological assessment of Asian Americans, and practical guidelines for such an assessment have been provided. Those working with patients of Asian descent are strongly encouraged to obtain information and understanding relevant to the particular individual through research and reading of materials related to the specific ethnic/cultural subgroup and through a careful interview that includes questions and discussion regarding cultural background and issues.

References

Alegado, D. (1987 September/October). Profile: U.S. Filipinos in the 1980s. *Katipunan*, 11.

American Psychological Association. (1993). Guidelines for providers of psychological services to ethnic, linguistic, and culturally diverse populations. *American Psychologist, 48*, 45–48.

American Psychological Association. (2002). Ethical principles of psychologists and code of conduct. *American Psychologist, 57*, 1060–1073.

Araneta, E. G. (1996). Psychiatric care of Filipino Americans. In A. Gaw (Ed.), *Culture, ethnicity, and mental illness* (pp. 377–411). Washington, DC: American Psychiatric Association.

Ardila, A. (1995). Directions of research in cross-cultural neuropsychology. *Journal of Clinical and Experimental Neuropsychology, 17*, 143–150.

Ardila, A., Rosselli, M., & Puente, A. (1994). *Neuropsychological evaluation of the Spanish-speaker.* New York: Plenum.

Army Individual Test Battery. (1944). *Manual of directions and scoring.* Washington, DC: War Department, Adjutant General's Office.

Artiola i Fortuny, L. (1997, August). *Spanish language normative studies: Very low education levels.* Paper presented at the American Psychological Association annual meeting, Scientific Program, Division of Clinical Neuropsychology (40), Chicago.

Artiola i Fortuny, L. (2003, February 5–8). *Clinical neuropsychology, low education, and illiteracy.* Paper presented at the International Neuropsychological Society 31st annual meeting, Honolulu, Hawaii.

Barnes, J. S., & Bennett, C. E. (2002). *The Asian population: 2000.* Washington, DC: U.S. Bureau of the Census.

Boehnlein, J. K., Leung, P. K., & Kinzie, J. D. (1997). Cambodian American families. In E. Lee (Ed.), *Working with Asian Americans: A guide for clinicians* (pp. 37–45). New York: Guilford.

D'Avanzo, C. E. (1997). Southeast Asians: Asian Pacific Americans at risk for substance misuse. *Substance Use & Misuse, 37*, 829–848.

Applied Neuropsychology
2004, Vol. 11, No. 1, 37–46

Acculturation, Reading Level, and Neuropsychological Test Performance Among African American Elders

Jennifer J. Manly, Desiree A. Byrd, and Pegah Touradji

*Cognitive Neuroscience Division, Taub Institute for Research
on Alzheimer's Disease and the Aging Brain, Department of Neurology,
Columbia University College of Physicians and Surgeons, New York, New York, USA*

Yaakov Stern

*Cognitive Neuroscience Division, Taub Institute for Research
on Alzheimer's Disease and the Aging Brain, Department of Neurology,
Columbia University College of Physicians and Surgeons, New York, New York, USA,
and Department of Psychiatry, Columbia University College of Physicians and Surgeons,
New York, New York, USA*

The independent effects of cultural and educational experience on neuropsychological test performance were examined among 503 nondemented African Americans ages 65 and older. Measures of cultural experience (acculturation) and quality of education (reading level) were administered. Reading level was the most influential predictor of cognitive test performance, even after accounting for age, sex, years of education, and acculturation level. Age had small but significant unique effects on most measures, especially word list learning. Years of education had independent effects on measures of verbal abstraction, fluency, and figure matching. More acculturated African Americans obtained higher scores on most measures; however, after accounting for age, years of education, sex, and reading level, the effect of acculturation was diminished. The results suggest that quality of education and cultural experience influence how older African Americans approach neuropsychological tasks; therefore, adjustment for these variables may improve specificity of neuropsychological measures.

Key words: quality of education, acculturation

Most studies of ethnic group differences in performance on intelligence, screening, and other neuropsychological measures have shown that discrepancies between scores of African Americans and Whites persist, despite matching groups on variables such as age, edu-

cation, sex, and income (reviewed in Manly & Jacobs, 2001; Nabors, Evans, & Strickland, 2000). These discrepancies attenuate the specificity of neuropsychological tests such that cognitively normal African Americans are more likely than Whites to be misdiagnosed as cognitively impaired (Ford-Booker et al., 1993; Klusman, Moulton, Hornbostle, Picano, & Beattie, 1991; Manly et al., 1998b; Stern et al., 1992; Welsh et al., 1995). Many investigators have concluded that separate neuropsychological test norms for African Americans and other ethnic groups are the solution to this problem (Ardila, 1995; Nabors et al., 2000; Wong, Strickland, Fletcher-Janzen, Ardila, & Reynolds, 2000).

Use of separate ethnic group norms most likely will reduce misdiagnosis of cognitive impairment among African Americans; however, there are significant disadvantages to this approach. Primarily, the use of sep-

This research was supported by federal grants AG16206 (J. Manly), AG07232 (R. Mayeux), the Alzheimer's Association, and the New York City Speakers Fund for Biomedical Research–Toward the Science of Patient Care. The authors thank Rosann Costa for her help with data management and Judes Fleurimont, Maria Gonzalez-Diaz, Cherita McDowell, Danurys Sanchez, Stacey Tuchin, and Wizdom Powell for their assistance with scheduling and interviewing participants.

Pegah Touradji is completing her postdoctorial fellowship at James A. Haley Veterans Hospital in Tampa, Florida.

Requests for reprints should be sent to Jennifer Manly, G.H. Sergievsky Center, 630 West 168th Street, P & S Box 16, New York, NY 10032. E-mail: jjm71@columbia.edu

arate norms may leave ethnic differences in test performance unexplained, unexamined, and thus not understood. Many authors (Helms, 1992; Neisser et al., 1996) have described how genetic or biological factors are often invoked to account for these unexplained differences. In contrast to the biological/genetic hypothesis, researchers in the 1970s began to propose that, because intelligence tests and other achievement measures incorrectly assumed a high level of literacy and equivalent school experiences, the tests were culturally biased against ethnic minorities and had unacceptable reliability and validity when used in these groups (Hilliard, 1979; Williams, 1971, 1974; van de Vijver, 1997). Helms argued that persisting test score discrepancies between African Americans and Whites reflect poor functional equivalence of cognitive tasks in the two ethnic groups. That is, measures developed in the majority culture may not assess the same cognitive ability in the same way when applied to African Americans. Early challenges to the biological/genetic hypotheses also focused on the ability of socioeconomic differences to explain ethnic differences in cognitive test performance. One of the first studies on quality of education and cognitive test performance showed that African American Army recruits schooled in northern states obtained higher average scores on the Army Alpha test than Whites schooled in southern states; furthermore, African Americans' scores increased for every year they stayed in northern cities (Klineberg, 1935). Still other investigators focused on measurement issues and held that, once socioeconomic variables were properly measured and accounted for, ethnic differences in IQ would disappear (Mercer, 1974).

Another major drawback underlying separate ethnic group norms is the assumption embedded in racial and ethnic classifications. Use of norms separated on the basis of race assumes that racial classifications are consistent and scientific. Because "Black," "African American," and "White" are social–political classifications as opposed to scientifically or genetically defined categories (Harrison, 1995; Smedley, 1999; D. Y. Wilkinson & King, 1987), it is unclear who should be included in normative studies for African Americans and to whom these norms should be applied. As the number of biracial and multiracial Americans increases, neuropsychologists would have to address how ethnic group norms would be applied to those with mixed heritage for whom traditional racial classifications are unclear or inappropriate. These complicated issues highlight the advantages of deconstructing race into the consistent, meaningful, and predictive variables that underlie the relationship between race and cognitive test performance.

As early as 1935, studies such as Klineberg's (1935) work with African American and White Army recruits demonstrated that specification of experiential, attitudinal, or behavioral variables that distinguish those belonging to different ethnic and racial groups and that also vary among people within an ethnic group may allow investigators to understand the underlying reasons for ethnic group differences in cognitive test performance. There is tremendous diversity in geographic, economic, and educational experiences, as well as level of exposure to majority culture, among African Americans. Current racial and ethnic classifications ignore this diversity. Our research group has begun to identify these within-group cultural factors, to measure them, and to explore their relationship to cognitive test performance. This investigational approach may illuminate factors that can explain ethnic group differences on cognitive tests. It also can inform us in the future regarding the development of measures of cognitive abilities that are salient within African American culture. The effect of these cultural and educational factors on cognitive test performance must be well understood before the development of "culture-fair" measures.

Level of acculturation was the first variable our research team used to operationalize within-group cultural variability. Previous studies have identified ideologies, beliefs, expectations, and attitudes as important components of acculturation, as well as cognitive and behavioral characteristics such as language and cognitive style (Berry, 1976; Moyerman & Forman, 1992; Negy & Woods, 1992; Padilla, 1980). Acculturation has traditionally been measured among immigrant groups such as Hispanics and Asian Americans; however, in 1994, Landrine and Klonoff (1994) reported the development of a reliable and valid measure of African American acculturation. This scale assesses traditional childhood experiences; religious beliefs and practices; preferences for African American music, media, and people; and preparation and consumption of traditional foods. When acculturation is measured, the association of cultural experience with cognitive test performance can be assessed, and hypotheses regarding test performance among people with lifestyles that are very dissimilar to the majority culture can be tested.

Previous research on Hispanic groups has shown a relationship between acculturation and performance on selected tests of the Halstead–Reitan Battery among college students (Arnold, Montgomery, Castaneda, & Longoria, 1994), as well as a relationship between years in the United States (a strong correlate of acculturation level) and perseverative errors on the Wisconsin Card Sorting Test (Artiola i Fortuny, Heaton, & Hermosillo, 1998). Three studies have explored the relationship of African American acculturation to cognitive test performance. Manly and colleagues (Manly et al., 1998) found that, among neurologically intact African Americans between the ages of 20 and 65, those who were less acculturated (more traditional) obtained lower scores on the Wechsler Adult Intelligence Scale–Revised (WAIS–R) Information subtest and the Boston Naming Test than more acculturated African Americans. Also in this study, differences in neuropsychological test scores between age, education, and disease-stage-matched HIV-positive African Americans and Whites were eliminated after controlling for acculturation level. Among elderly African Americans living in Jacksonville, Florida, acculturation accounted for a significant amount of variance in Verbal IQ (as measured by the WAIS–R), Boston Naming Test, and delayed recall of stories from the Wechsler Memory Scale–Revised (Lucas, 1998). A recent study found that, among African American traumatic brain injury patients, those who were less acculturated obtained lower scores on a neuropsychological test battery overall and specifically on the Grooved Pegboard and WAIS–R Block Design and achieved a lower number of categories on the Wisconsin Card Sorting Test (Kennepohl, Shore, Nabors, & Hanks, in press). A preliminary study among elderly, nondemented African American residents of northern Manhattan revealed that those who were more traditional (less acculturated), as assessed by the African American Acculturation Scale (AAAS), obtained lower scores on measures of figure memory, naming, repetition, and figure matching (Manly et al., 1998a). Taken together, investigations of acculturation suggest that there are cultural differences within elders of the same ethnicity that relate to neuropsychological measures of verbal skills, executive function, and psychomotor speed and that accounting for acculturation (in addition to age, years of education, and sex) may help improve the ability of certain neuropsychological tests to detect subtle impairment.

Schooling is another aspect of cultural experience that has been proven to have significant effects on neuropsychological test performance, regardless of race or ethnicity (Adams, Boake, & Crain, 1982; Heaton, Grant, & Matthews, 1986; Lezak, 1995). However, in the United States, there is a great deal of discordance between years of education and quality of education; this is especially true among African Americans. Factors such as whether African Americans attended school before or after the Supreme Court's 1954 Brown v. Board of Education decision banning segregation in public schools, unequal distribution of educational funds, variable teacher education, shorter length of school year, and lower attendance because of required work had a profound effect on the quality of education received by African Americans (Anderson, 1988; Margo, 1990). These variables are among the multiple factors that have been found to explain the differences between African Americans and Whites on achievement measures and other outcomes such as wage earnings (Hanushek, 1989; Hedges, Laine, & Greenwald, 1994; O'Neill, 1990). Previous studies have demonstrated that African Americans had reading skills that were significantly below their self-reported education level (Albert & Teresi, 1999; Baker, Johnson, Velli, & Wiley, 1996; Manly, Jacobs, Touradji, Small, & Stern, 2002). Therefore, disparate school experiences and resulting different bases of problem-solving strategies, knowledge, familiarity, and practice could explain why some African Americans obtain lower scores on cognitive measures even after controlling for years of education. Statistical control for years of education may be an inadequate or inappropriate method for equating racial groups on educational experience because quality of education differs so dramatically between African Americans and Whites, as well as within African Americans (e.g., depending on whether they were educated in segregated or integrated schools or in rural or urban settings; Kaufman, Cooper, & McGee, 1997; Loewenstein, Arguelles, Arguelles, & Linn-Fuentes, 1994).

Our research group recently reported a study that sought to determine whether discrepancies in quality of education could explain differences in cognitive test scores between African American and White elders matched on years of education (Manly et al., 2002). A comprehensive neuropsychological battery was administered to a sample of nondemented African American and non-Hispanic White participants in an epidemiological study of normal aging and dementia in the northern Manhattan community. The Reading Recognition subtest from the Wide Range Achievement Test–Version 3 (WRAT–3) was used as an estimate of quality of education. African American elders obtained significantly lower scores than Whites on measures of word list learning and memory, figure memory, abstract reasoning, fluency, and visuospatial skill, even though the groups were matched on years of education. However, after adjusting the scores for WRAT–3 reading score, the overall effect of race was greatly reduced, and racial differences on all tests (except category fluency and a drawing measure) became nonsignificant.

Reading score also attenuated the effect of race after accounting for an estimate of test wiseness. This finding suggests that years of education is an inadequate measure of the educational experience among multicultural elders and that adjusting for quality of education may improve the specificity of certain neuropsychological measures across racial groups.

The investigation reported here was an attempt to determine the role of age, sex, years of education, quality of education (as operationalized by reading level), and acculturation on neuropsychological test performance among African American elders. Our previous research (Manly et al., 1999; Manly et al., 2002; Manly et al., 1998) indicated that each of these variables would account for a significant amount of variance on performance on cognitive measures that tapped both verbal and nonverbal functions. However, because acculturation and reading level had not yet been measured in the same sample, it was unclear whether each would contribute uniquely to the prediction of cognitive test performance. Nevertheless, it was expected that elders with a high quality of education (and thus high reading levels) would obtain higher scores on neuropsychological measures of nonverbal memory, abstraction, naming, letter fluency, repetition, comprehension, and visuospatial skill than elders with a low quality of education and reading levels. Furthermore, it was hypothesized that reading level would be the strongest predictor of these cognitive test scores and thus would account for significant, unique variance in test scores when years of education, age, sex, and acculturation were entered into the model. With regard to cultural experience, it was expected that more acculturated African American elders would obtain higher scores on measures of figure recognition, verbal abstraction, naming, and figure matching than less acculturated elders. Acculturation was predicted to be a significant predictor of performance on these measures, albeit a weaker predictor than reading level.

Method

Research Participants

The sample was selected from participants in the Washington Heights–Inwood Columbia Aging Project (WHICAP), a community-based, epidemiological study of dementia in the ethnically diverse neighborhoods of northern Manhattan, New York. WHICAP longitudinally follows a sample of elderly Medicare recipients residing in selected census tracts of Washington/Hamilton Heights and Inwood. The population from which participants were drawn consists of people from several different countries of origin and represents three broadly defined ethnic categories (i.e., Hispanic, African American, and non-Hispanic White).

Inclusion and exclusion criteria. All potential participants were aged 65 and older and completed the neuropsychological battery in English. Participants were included if they self-identified their race as Black/African American and their "ethnicity" as non-Hispanic according to the 1997 revisions to the Office of Management and Budget's standards for data on race and ethnicity, which was used by the 2000 U.S. Census. Approximately 10% of WHICAP participants who described themselves as non-Hispanic Black were born in Jamaica, other Caribbean Islands such as Haiti, or Central America; the sample reported here was limited to African American elders born in the United States and for whom English was their first and primary language. Potential participants were excluded if they had a history of Parkinson's disease, stroke, head injury with loss of consciousness, alcohol or substance abuse, history of mental illness such as schizophrenia, or current major depression. Only WHICAP participants who showed no neurological or functional signs of dementia were included in the analyses reported here. This determination was made on the basis of a physician's clinical examination, which included a rating of daily functioning (see Procedure later in this article). The physician's diagnosis was used as a "gold standard" for the absence of dementia because the neurological assessment was made independent of the participant's performance on the neuropsychological battery.

Medical evaluation. A physician recorded medical history and medications in a semistructured format. Neurological and brief physical examinations were performed, including assessment of extrapyramidal signs. Functional status was measured using Part 1 of the Blessed Dementia Rating Scale (Blessed, Tomlinson, & Roth, 1968) and the Schwab and England rating scale of activities of daily living (Boller, Mizutani, Roessmann, & Gambetti, 1980). From this information, the physician determined whether the participant met criteria for delirium or dementia using the *Diagnostic and Statistical Manual of Mental Disorders 3rd. ed., Revised* (American Psychiatric Association, 1987) criteria.

Procedure

Neuropsychological battery. The evaluation included measures of learning, memory, orientation, abstract reasoning, language, and visuospatial ability. Specific ability areas and tests administered included verbal list learning and memory using the Selective Reminding Test (SRT; Buschke & Fuld, 1974); nonverbal memory from the multiple-choice version of the Benton Visual Retention Test (BVRT; Benton, 1955); orientation items from the Mini Mental State Examination (MMSE; Folstein, Folstein, & McHugh, 1975); verbal reasoning using the Similarities subtest of the WAIS–R (Wechsler, 1981); nonverbal reasoning from the Identities and Oddities subtest of the Mattis Dementia Rating Scale (DRS; Mattis, 1976); naming using a 15-item version of the Boston Naming Test (Kaplan, Goodglass, & Weintraub, 1983); letter fluency from the Controlled Word Association Test (Benton & Hamsher, 1976); category fluency using procedures from the Boston Diagnostic Aphasia Examination (BDAE) and the categories of animals, food, and clothing (Goodglass & Kaplan, 1983); repetition of high-frequency phrases from the BDAE (Goodglass et al., 1983); auditory comprehension of the first 6 items of the Complex Ideational Material subtest of the BDAE (Goodglass et al., 1983); visuoconstruction using the Rosen Drawing Test (Rosen, 1981); and visuoperceptual skills as assessed by multiple-choice matching of figures from the BVRT (Benton, 1955).

Reading level.   Reading level was measured using the Reading Recognition subtest from the WRAT–3 (G. S. Wilkinson, 1993). Participants were asked to name letters and pronounce words out of context. The words are listed in order of decreasing familiarity and increasing phonological complexity. Consistent with the standard instructions for administration, a basal of 5 correct and a ceiling of 10 incorrect was used.

Acculturation.   Each participant's level of acculturation was measured using the short form of the AAAS (Landrine & Klonoff, 1994, 1995). Each of the 33 items assesses traditions, values, beliefs, assumptions, and practices found in African American culture. The short-form AAAS measures acculturation across 10 dimensions: preference for African American music, arts, and people; religious beliefs and practices; traditional foods; traditional childhood experiences; superstitions; interracial attitudes/cultural mistrust; falling out (knowledge and experience of a folk disorder); traditional games; and family values. The four AAAS subscales that accounted for the most variance in the Landrine and Klonoff (1995) standardization sample were preferences (e.g., "Most of the music I lis-

ten to is by Black artists"); foods and food practices (e.g., "Sometimes, I cook ham hocks"); religious beliefs and practices (e.g., "I am currently a member of a Black church"); and traditional childhood experiences (e.g., "I grew up in a mostly Black neighborhood"). Landrine and Klonoff (1995) found that the AAAS-33 could distinguish well between African Americans and non-African Americans, had acceptable concurrent validity, split-half reliability of $r = .77$, and an internal consistency reliability (Cronbach's alpha) of $r = .81$ among African Americans. Scores on the subscales were not significantly related to social class, education, or social class of origin in the original standardization sample. In its original version, the AAAS is a self-administered, paper-and-pencil survey. To accommodate older participants who had poor vision or low levels of literacy, the measure was slightly modified from the published version such that the scale was administered in a face-to-face interview and the original Likert scale was simplified. In this slightly modified version, participants chose one of the following responses to each item: "I disagree/This is not at all true of me," "Sort of agree/This is sort of true of me," or "I strongly agree/This is definitely true of me." Our modified version has an internal consistency reliability (Cronbach's alpha) of .71 and a Guttman split-half reliability of $r = .61$ (Powell, Tuchin, Touradji, & Manly, 2000). In the analyses presented here, the summary score from the AAAS was used to represent acculturation level.

Statistical Methods

Simple bivariate correlation analyses and *t* tests were used to determine the strength of the relationships among the predictors: age, sex, years of education, acculturation (total score on the AAAS), and WRAT–3 reading level.

The next set of analyses used simple regression models to determine the relationships between each of the five predictor variables (age, sex, years of education, total score on the AAAS, and WRAT–3 reading level) and performance on each of the neuropsychological tests. The 13 measures used as dependent variables were total raw scores for immediate recall and delayed recall from the SRT, BVRT matching and recognition score, items correct on the MMSE Orientation, 15-item Boston Naming, BDAE repetition, BDAE comprehension, Mattis Identities and Oddities, number correct on the Rosen Drawing Test, raw score on WAIS–R Similarities, and mean number of words generated over three 60-sec trials for category and letter fluency. Each of these 13 dependent variables was predicted by each of the 5 dependent variables, which were entered into the equation alone. Effect size is reported as the proportion of variance in each test score accounted for by the predictor variable.

Finally, multiple regression was used to determine the independent contributions of age, sex, years of education, acculturation level, and reading score to the prediction of each neuropsychological test score. In each regression equation, age, years of education, sex, acculturation, and reading level were entered together as predictors of neuropsychological test performance. The partial regression coefficients for each of the predictors were examined to determine which variables accounted for unique and significant amounts of variance in each cognitive test score. Alpha for all analyses was set at $p <$ .01 to strike a balance between the likelihood of committing Type I and Type II errors.

Results

Sample Characteristics

A total of 554 nondemented, English-speaking, American-born, non-Hispanic Black WHICAP participants had complete neuropsychological evaluations, WRAT–3 data, and neurological exams. Fifty-one participants were excluded because of a history of stroke ($n = 17$), head injury ($n = 8$), drug or alcohol abuse ($n = 5$), or psychiatric history ($n = 23$). Some patients had more than one exclusionary condition.

The remaining 503 African American elders had a mean age of 76.2 years ($SD = 6.1$), and 75% were women. Average years of education was 11.4 years ($SD = 3.7$) and ranged from 0 to 20 years. WRAT–3 reading subtest scores ranged from 13 (0–third-grade reading level) to 56 (post-high school reading level), with a mean of 42.2 ($SD = 8.1$).

Correlations Between Demographics, Acculturation, and Reading Level

The correlations between the primary independent variables are shown in Table 1. The correlations between these variables, although significant, indicate that the variables reflect constructs that are not multicollinear. Older African Americans had fewer years of education relative to younger African Americans. As expected, African Americans with more years of education had higher scores on the WRAT–3 reading subtest and were more acculturated. Higher scores on the WRAT–3 reading subtest were associated with reports of less traditional (more acculturated) lifestyle as re-

Table 1. *Correlations Between Independent Variables*

	Age	Years of Education	AAAS Total
Age	1.00		
Years of education	−.15*	1.00	
AAAS total	−.07	−.24*	1.00
WRAT–3 reading	−.08	.59*	−.28*

Note: AAAS = African American Acculturation Scale; WRAT–3 = Wide-Range Achievement Test–Version 3.
*$p < .001$.

ported on the AAAS. T tests showed that elderly African American women in this sample were significantly older than elderly African American men, $t(501) =$ 3.77, $p < .001$.

Demographics, Acculturation, Reading Level, and Neuropsychological Test Performance

Table 2 shows the proportion of variance accounted for by each of the predictor variables in simple regression equations predicting each of the neuropsychological test scores. Sex was not a significant predictor of performance on any of the measures, accounting for no more than 0.5% of variance in any of the scores. Age accounted for 1% to 11% of variance in neuropsychological test scores, with its strongest effects on SRT total recall score. Elders with fewer years of school obtained lower scores on the measures; the effect size of years of education ranged from 2% to 32%. Acculturation was a significant but weak predictor of test scores, accounting for no more than 6% of variance on any measure. Finally, WRAT–3 reading score had strong, positive relationships with performance, accounting for 3% to 40% of the variance in test scores.

Multiple regression analyses revealed that reading level was the strongest independent predictor of most measures in the neuropsychological battery ($p < .001$ for all). Among the independent variables, reading level accounted for the largest proportion of unique variance on all but 5 of the 13 variables: SRT total and delayed recall, Mattis DRS Identities and Oddities, category fluency, and BVRT matching. In contrast, although years of education had an independent effect on 6 of the measures, it did not uniquely contribute to the prediction of delayed recall of a word list, orientation, nonverbal abstract reasoning, naming, repetition, comprehension, or drawing.

Age was a significant, independent predictor of scores on all measures except orientation, repetition, and comprehension ($p < .005$ for all). Acculturation

Table 2. *Proportion of Variance (R²) in Neuropsychological Test Scores Accounted for by Demographics, Acculturation, and Reading Level*

Test	Sex[a]	Age	Years of Education	Acculturation	WRAT–3 Reading
Learning/memory					
SRT total recall	.001	.119	.166	.025	.189
SRT delayed recall	.001	.070	.091	.011[b]	.105
BVRT recognition memory	.004	.059	.156	.029	.211
Orientation					
MMSE orientation	.004	.012[b]	.020	.002[b]	.033
Abstract reasoning					
WAIS–R similarities raw	.005	.062	.319	.060	.386
DRS identities and oddities	.005	.045	.077	.003[b]	.088
Language					
Boston Naming	.002	.025	.148	.048	.316
Letter fluency	.002	.046	.216	.030	.401
Category fluency	.000	.070	.184	.028	.184
BDAE repetition	.004	.010[b]	.057	.028	.095
BDAE comprehension	.003	.012[b]	.096	.017	.137
Visuospatial ability					
Rosen Drawing	.001	.036	.071	.039	.116
BVRT matching	.001	.058	.139	.038	.156

Note: R^2 is the proportion of variance in neuropsychological test score accounted for by the independent variable in a simple linear regression. WRAT–3 = Wide Range Achievement Test–Version 3; SRT = Selective Reminding Test; BVRT = Benton Visual Retention Test; MMSE = Mini Mental State Examination; WAIS–R = Wechsler Adult Intelligence Scale–Revised; DRS = Dementia Rating Scale; BDAE = Boston Diagnostic Aphasia Examination. All values shown had a *p* value less than .01 with the following exceptions.
[a]None of the R^2 values for the effect of sex were significant below the .01 level. [b]These values did not reach significance.

contributed significantly to the prediction of scores on only Rosen Drawing; however, there was a trend for more acculturated African American elders to obtain higher scores on the WAIS–R Similarities subtest ($sr^2 = .01, p = .03$) and delayed figure recognition ($sr^2 = .01, p = .02$) than more traditional (less acculturated) elders. Sex was not a significant unique predictor of performance on any of the cognitive measures.

Discussion

The results show that, among African American elders, age, years of education, acculturation level, and reading ability have significant, independent effects on neuropsychological test scores across several cognitive domains. The magnitude of the association between reading level and test performance was greatest on measures of verbal abstraction, naming, and phonemic fluency. Furthermore, reading level was consistently a significant unique predictor of test performance across cognitive domains. Older African Americans obtained significantly lower scores on several measures, especially verbal word list learning; however, the independent effect of age on test score was weak relative to the association between reading level and test score. Elders with fewer years of school obtained lower scores on all measures; but again, in the context of the other demo-graphic variables such as acculturation and reading level, the association of years of education with test performance was diminished. Finally, acculturation level was a unique predictor of only drawing skill. These findings support the use of within-group cultural and educational variables to adjust expectations of test performance among African American elders.

Hypotheses regarding quality of education (as operationalized by reading level) were based on our previous work with elders with no formal education (Manly et al., 1999), as well as a study that used the WRAT–3 to explain differences in test performance between African American and White elders (Manly et al., 2002). These hypotheses were partially confirmed. African Americans with lower reading levels obtained lower scores on measures of figure memory, verbal abstraction, naming, letter fluency, comprehension, phrase repetition, and visuospatial skill; these effects were independent of acculturation, age, years of education, and sex. However, contrary to our original hypotheses, reading level also had a significant unique effect on learning and delayed recall scores from the SRT, orientation, a measure of nonverbal abstraction (Identities and Oddities from the DRS), as well as words generated within a particular category (animals, foods, and clothing). Nevertheless, the effect sizes of reading level for these measures (2% to 7% of the variance of the test scores uniquely accounted for by WRAT–3) were much smaller than the effect sizes of reading level for other measures such as verbal abstraction, naming, and letter fluency (ranging from 5% to 26%).

These results add to the literature, suggesting that reading level is a more sensitive proxy for educational experience than years of education among African American elders. However, educational quality is only one of many variables that may influence reading recognition scores, including general (native) cognitive ability, reading experience obtained through access to books in the home or as a result of occupational demands, and test wiseness. Future study will explore the relationship of WRAT–3 reading score to other measures of educational quality such as per-student expenditures, teacher salaries, and length of school year. Regardless of the abilities and experiences that determine reading level, this skill appears to be the strongest predictor of cognitive test performance among African American elders.

It was hypothesized that acculturation level would be a unique predictor of performance on certain cognitive measures; however, this hypothesis was largely unsupported by the data. African American elders who were more acculturated obtained higher scores than traditional African American elders on all measures except delayed recall of a word list, orientation, and nonverbal abstraction. However, once other demographic variables and reading level were entered into the model, the unique effect of acculturation was significant only for Rosen Drawing, in which AAAS score accounted for only 2% of the variance.

The association of cognitive test performance with acculturation level and reading skill could be explained by other cognitive and noncognitive factors that have a direct influence on test performance. For example, acculturation level may reflect the salience that a particular task has in everyday life. Traditional cognitive measures are based within a dominant culture that emphasizes individualism, detail, and speeded performance, whereas traditional African Americans are more likely to ascribe to a belief system that is spiritually based and holistic and that emphasizes interpersonal relationships (Asante, 1990; Boykin, Jagers, Ellison, & Albury, 1997; Shade, 1991). Less acculturated elders, as well as African Americans who attended poorly funded, segregated schools, may not be as "testwise" or as proficient in the implicit and explicit language of neuropsychological assessment. Acculturation and reading level also may reflect the influence of racial socialization on motivation or attitude toward testing. For example, African American children with higher levels of cultural mistrust obtained lower scores

on cognitive measures when assessed by a White examiner (Terrell, Terrell, & Taylor, 1981).

The complete range of cognitive skills and learning strategies of ethnic minorities may not be adequately tapped by standard cognitive tasks. Perhaps traditional neuropsychological tests simply do not elicit the full potential of all African Americans and other ethnic minority groups. Assessment of these yet-unmeasured strengths could be the best way to detect subtle neurocognitive dysfunction among ethnic minorities. Evidence that supports this possibility is derived from studies demonstrating that, when test stimuli are more culturally pertinent to the experiences of African Americans, performance improves (Hayles, 1991). Prior research indicates that African Americans obtain higher scaled scores on measures of divergent thinking or creativity than on traditional measures of general information or verbal abstraction (Price-Williams & Ramirez, 1977; Torrance, 1971). In addition, some research shows that, in contrast to reports of lower African American performance on memory tests with verbal and figural stimuli, African Americans obtain higher scores on measures of facial recognition (both White and Black faces) than Whites (Barkowitz & Brigham, 1982; Golby, Gabrieli, Chiao, & Eberhardt, 2001), suggesting increased salience or experience with human face processing among African Americans. These studies point to several alternative ways in which neuropsychological measures can be used to assess cognitive abilities that are salient within African American culture.

Studies of the effect of within-group cultural and educational factors on test performance can serve as hypothesis generators for in-depth study of the effect of these variables on specific cognitive functions. Once we understand the nature of the relationship between cultural and educational variables and test performance, we may be able to more successfully develop tests that are specific and sensitive to neurocognitive impairment among African Americans.

References

Adams, R. L., Boake, C., & Crain, C. (1982). Bias in a neuropsychological test classification related to age, education and ethnicity. *Journal of Consulting and Clinical Psychology, 50,* 143–145.

Albert, S. M., & Teresi, J. A. (1999). Reading ability, education, and cognitive status assessment among older adults in Harlem, New York City. *American Journal of Public Health, 89,* 95–97.

American Psychiatric Association. (1987). *Diagnostic and Statistical Manual of Mental Disorders* (3rd ed., revised). Washington, DC: Author.

Anderson, J. D. (1988). *The education of Blacks in the South, 1860–1935.* Chapel Hill: University of North Carolina Press.

Ardila, A. (1995). Directions of research in cross-cultural neuropsychology. *Journal of Clinical and Experimental Neuropsychology, 17,* 143–150.

Arnold, B. R., Montgomery, G. T., Castaneda, I., & Longoria, R. (1994). Acculturation and performance of Hispanics on selected Halstead-Reitan neuropsychological tests. *Assessment, 1,* 239–248.

Artiola i Fortuny, L., Heaton, R. K., & Hermosillo, D. (1998). Neuropsychological comparisons of Spanish-speaking participants from the U.S.–Mexico border region versus Spain. *Journal of the International Neuropsychological Society, 4,* 363–379.

Asante, M. K., & Asante, A. K. W. (1990). *African culture and the rhythms of unity.* Trenton, NJ: Africa World Press.

Baker, F. M., Johnson, J. T., Velli, S. A., & Wiley, C. (1996). Congruence between education and reading levels of older persons. *Psychiatric Services, 47,* 194–196.

Barkowitz, P., & Brigham, J. C. (1982). Recognition of faces: Own-race, incentive, and time-delay. *Journal of Applied Social Psychology, 12,* 225–268.

Benton, A. L. (1955). *The Visual Retention Test.* New York: Psychological Corporation.

Benton, A. L., & Hamsher, K. D. (1976). *Multilingual aphasia examination.* Iowa City: University of Iowa Press.

Berry, J. W. (1976). *Human ecology and cognitive style.* New York: Sage-Halsted.

Blessed, G., Tomlinson, B. E., & Roth, M. (1968). The association between quantitative measures of senile change in the cerebral grey matter of elderly subjects. *British Journal of Psychology, 114,* 797–811.

Boller, F., Mizutani, T., Roessmann, U., & Gambetti, P. (1980). Parkinson's disease, dementia, and Alzheimer's disease: Clinicopathological correlations. *Annals of Neurology, 1,* 329–335.

Boykin, W., Jagers, R. J., Ellison, C. M., & Albury, A. (1997). Communalism: Conceptualization and measurement of an Afrocultural social orientation. *Journal of Black Studies, 27,* 409–418.

Buschke, H., & Fuld, P. A. (1974). Evaluating storage, retention, and retrieval in disordered memory and learning. *Neurology, 24,* 1019–1025.

Folstein, M. F., Folstein, S. E., & McHugh, P. R. (1975). "Mini-Mental State": A practical method for grading the cognitive state of patients for the clinician. *Journal of Psychiatric Research, 12,* 189–198.

Ford-Booker, P., Campbell, A., Combs, S., Lewis, S., Ocampo, C., Brown, A., et al. (1993). The predictive accuracy of neuropsychological tests in a normal population of African Americans. *Journal of Clinical and Experimental Neuropsychology, 15,* 64.

Golby, A. J., Gabrieli, J. D., Chiao, J. Y., & Eberhardt, J. L. (2001). Differential responses in the fusiform region to same-race and other-race faces. *Nature Neuroscience, 4,* 845–850.

Goodglass, H., & Kaplan, E. (1983). *The assessment of aphasia and related disorders* (2nd ed.). Philadelphia: Lea & Febiger.

Hanushek, E. (1989). The impact of differential expenditures on school performance. *Educational Researcher, 18*(4), 45–51.

Harrison, F. V. (1995). The persistent power of "race" in the cultural and political economy of racism. *Annual Review of Anthropology, 24,* 47–74.

Hayles, V. R. (1991). African American strengths: A survey of empirical findings. In R. L. Jones (Ed.), *Black psychology* (3rd ed., pp. 379–400). Berkeley, CA: Cobb & Henry Publishers.

Heaton, R. K., Grant, I., & Matthews, C. G. (1986). Differences in neuropsychological test performance associated with age, education, and sex. In I. Grant & K. M. Adams (Eds.), *Neuropsychological assessment of neuropsychiatric disorders* (1st ed., pp. 100–120). New York: Oxford University Press.

Hedges, L. V., Laine, R. D., & Greenwald, R. (1994). Does money matter? A meta-analysis of studies of the effects of differential school inputs on student outcomes. *Educational Researcher, 23*(3), 5–14.

Helms, J. E. (1992). Why is there no study of cultural equivalence in standardized cognitive ability testing? *American Psychologist, 47,* 1083–1101.

Hilliard, A. G. (1979). Standardization and cultural bias impediments to the scientific study and validation of "intelligence." *Journal of Research and Development in Education, 12,* 47–58.

Kaplan, E., Goodglass, H., & Weintraub, S. (1983). *Boston Naming Test.* Philadelphia: Lea & Febiger.

Kaufman, J. S., Cooper, R. S., & McGee, D. L. (1997). Socioeconomic status and health in blacks and whites: The problem of residual confounding and the resilience of race. *Epidemiology, 8,* 621–628.

Kennepohl, S., Shore, D., Nabors, N., & Hanks, R. (in press). African American acculturation and neuropsychological test performance following traumatic brain injury. *Journal of the International Neuropsychological Society.*

Klineberg, O. (1935). *Race differences.* New York: Harper & Brothers.

Klusman, L. E., Moulton, J. M., Hornbostle, L. K., Picano, J. J., & Beattie, M. T. (1991). Neuropsychological abnormalities in asymptomatic HIV seropositive military personnel. *Journal of Neuropsychological and Clinical Neurosciences, 3,* 422–428.

Landrine, H., & Klonoff, E. A. (1994). The African American Acculturation Scale: Development, reliability, and validity. *Journal of Black Psychology, 20,* 104–127.

Landrine, H., & Klonoff, E. A. (1995). The African American Acculturation Scale II: Cross-validation and short form. *Journal of Black Psychology, 21,* 124–152.

Lezak, M. D. (1995). *Neuropsychological assessment* (3rd ed.). New York: Oxford University Press.

Loewenstein, D. A., Arguelles, T., Arguelles, S., & Linn-Fuentes, P. (1994). Potential cultural bias in the neuropsychological assessment of the older adult. *Journal of Clinical and Experimental Neuropsychology, 16,* 623–629.

Lucas, J. A. (1998). Acculturation and neuropsychological test performance in elderly African Americans. *Journal of the International Neuropsychological Society, 4,* 77.

Manly, J. J., & Jacobs, D. M. (2001). Future directions in neuropsychological assessment with African Americans. In F. R. Ferraro (Ed.), *Minority and cross-cultural aspects of neuropsychological assessment* (pp. 79–96). Lisse, Netherlands: Swets & Zeitlinger.

Manly, J. J., Jacobs, D. M., Sano, M., Bell, K., Merchant, C. A., Small, S. A., et al. (1998a). African American acculturation and neuropsychological test performance among nondemented community elders. *Journal of the International Neuropsychological Society, 4,* 77.

Manly, J. J., Jacobs, D. M., Sano, M., Bell, K., Merchant, C. A., Small, S. A., et al. (1998b). Cognitive test performance among nondemented elderly African Americans and Whites. *Neurology, 50,* 1238–1245.

Manly, J. J., Jacobs, D. M., Sano, M., Bell, K., Merchant, C. A., Small, S. A., et al. (1999). Effect of literacy on neuropsychological test performance in nondemented, education-matched elders. *Journal of the International Neuropsychological Society, 5,* 191–202.

Manly, J. J., Jacobs, D. M., Touradji, P., Small, S. A., & Stern, Y. (2002). Reading level attenuates differences in neuropsychological test performance between African American and White elders. *Journal of the International Neuropsychological Society, 8,* 341–348.

Manly, J. J., Miller, S. W., Heaton, R. K., Byrd, D., Reilly, J., Velasquez, R. J., et al. (1998). The effect of African American acculturation on neuropsychological test performance in normal and HIV positive individuals. *Journal of the International Neuropsychological Society, 4,* 291–302.

Margo, R. A. (1990). *Race and schooling in the South, 1880–1950: An economic history.* Chicago: University of Chicago Press.

Mattis, S. (1976). Mental status examination for organic mental syndrome in the elderly patient. In L. Bellak & T. B. Karasu (Eds.), *Geriatric psychiatry* (pp. 77–121). New York: Grune & Stratton

Mercer, J. R. (1974). *Labeling the mentally retarded: Clinical and social system perspectives on mental retardation.* Berkeley: University of California Press.

Moyerman, D. R., & Forman, B. D. (1992). Acculturation and adjustment—a meta-analytic study. *Hispanic Journal of Behavioral Sciences, 14,* 163–200.

Nabors, N. A., Evans, J. D., & Strickland, T. L. (2000). Neuropsychological assessment and intervention with African Americans. In E. Fletcher-Janzen, T. L. Strickland, & C. Reynolds (Eds.), *Handbook of cross-cultural neuropsychology* (pp. 31–42). New York: Kluwer Academic.

Negy, C., & Woods, D. J. (1992). The importance of acculturation in understanding research with Hispanic-Americans. *Hispanic Journal of Behavioral Sciences, 14,* 224–247.

Neisser, U., Boodoo, G., Bouchard, T. J. J., Boykin, A. W., Brody, N., Ceci, S. J., et al. (1996). Intelligence: Knowns and unknowns. *American Psychologist, 51,* 77–101.

O'Neill, J. (1990). The role of human capitol in earning differences between Black and White men. *Journal of Economic Perspectives, 4,* 25–45.

Padilla, A. M. (1980). *Acculturation: Theory, models, and some new findings.* Boulder, CO: Westview for the American Association for the Advancement of Science.

Powell, W. A., Tuchin, S. R., Touradji, P., & Manly, J. J. (2000). *African American acculturation among nondemented elders.* Paper presented at the annual meeting of the American Psychological Association, Washington, DC.

Price-Williams, D. R., & Ramirez, M. (1977). Divergent thinking, cultural deficiencies and civilizations. *Journal of Social Psychology, 103,* 3–11.

Rosen, W. (1981). *The Rosen Drawing Test.* Bronx, NY: Veterans Administration Medical Center.

Shade, B. J. (1991). African American patterns of cognition. In R. L. Jones (Ed.), *Black psychology* (3rd ed., pp. 231–247). Berkeley, CA: Cobb & Henry Publishers.

Smedley, A. (1999). *Race in North America: Origin and evolution of a worldview.* (2nd ed.) Boulder, CO: Westview.

Stern, Y., Andrews, H., Pittman, J., Sano, M., Tatemichi, T., Lantigua, R., et al. (1992). Diagnosis of dementia in a heterogeneous population. Development of a neuropsychological paradigm-based diagnosis of dementia and quantified correction for the effects of education. *Archives of Neurology, 49,* 453–460.

Terrell, F., Terrell, S. L., & Taylor, J. (1981). Effects of race of examiner and cultural mistrust on the WAIS performance of Black students. *Journal of Consulting and Clinical Psychology, 49,* 750–751.

Torrance, E. P. (1971). Are the Torrance Tests of Creative Thinking biased against or in favor of "disadvantaged" groups? *Gifted Child Quarterly, 15,* 75–80

van de Vijver, F. (1997). Meta-analysis of cross-cultural comparisons of cognitive test performance. *Journal of Cross-Cultural Psychology, 28,* 678–709.

Wechsler, D. (1981). *Wechsler Adult Intelligence Scale–Revised.* New York: Psychological Corporation.

Welsh, K. A., Fillenbaum, G., Wilkinson, W., Heyman, A., Mohs, R. C., Stern, Y., et al. (1995). Neuropsychological test performance in African American and white patients with Alzheimer's disease. *Neurology, 45,* 2207–2211.

Wilkinson, G. S. (1993). *Wide Range Achievement Test 3—Administration manual.* Wilmington, DE: Jastak Associates.

Wilkinson, D. Y., & King, G. (1987). Conceptual and methodological issues in the use of race as a variable: Policy implications. *Milbank Quarterly, 65,* 56–71.

Williams, R. L. (1971). Abuses and misuses in testing black children. *Counseling Psychologist, 2,* 62–73.

Williams, R. L. (1974). Scientific racism and IQ: The silent mugging of the black community. *Psychology Today, 7,* 32–41.

Wong, T. M., Strickland, T. L., Fletcher-Janzen, E., Ardila, A., & Reynolds, C. R. (2000). Theoretical and practical issues in the neuropsychological assessment and treatment of culturally dissimilar patients. In E. Fletcher-Janzen, T. L. Strickland, & C. R. Reynolds (Eds.), *Handbook of cross-cultural neuropsychology* (pp. 3–18). New York: Kluwer Academic.

Applied Neuropsychology
2004, Vol. 11, No. 1, 47–53

Differences in Neuropsychological Performance Associated With Ethnicity in Children With HIV-1 Infection: Preliminary Findings

Antolin M. Llorente

*Department of Pediatrics, University of Maryland School of Medicine,
Baltimore, Maryland, USA,*

and Mount Washington Pediatric Hospital, Baltimore, Maryland, USA

Marie Turcich

*Department of Pediatrics, Baylor College of Medicine and Texas Children's Hospital,
Houston, Texas, USA*

Kelly A. Lawrence

Department of Psychology, Loyola College, Baltimore, Maryland, USA

This study investigated the relationship between ethnicity (African American and European American) and neuropsychological performance in two specific neuropsychological domains (language and speed of information processing) in a group of HIV-1+ children. The Expressive One-Word Picture Vocabulary Test–Revised and the Rapid Color Naming subtest of the Comprehensive Test of Phonological Processing were administered to 5- to 7-year-old children (n = 22) as part of a comprehensive research or clinical protocol. African American children scored lower than European American children (p < .05) on both procedures. The observed performance difference emerged despite the fact that there were no group differences in age, immunologic clinical categories, intellect, level of maternal education, or CD4+ percentage and after using stringent exclusionary criteria, including history of enrollment in special education services and the presence of other chronic medical conditions. The implications of such findings are discussed within biological and demographic frameworks.

Key words: ethnicity, children, HIV-1 infection, emerging language, information processing

Children infected with HIV-1 may exhibit neurological (Belman et al., 1985), neurodevelopmental (Chase et al., 2000), and neuropsychological (Brouwers, Wolters, & Civitello, 1998; Llorente, LoPresti, & Satz, 1997) abnormalities. HIV-1-related neurocognitive manifestations may be predictive of mortality during infancy and early childhood (Llorente et al., 2003) and an independent risk factor for mortality during adult-

hood (Ellis et al., 1997). The cause of these anomalies and morbidity has been attributed to underlying neuropathology (Epstein et al., 1985; Sharer et al., 1990), damage that appears to be directly related to the effects of this virus on neuronal substrates (cf. Lyman et al., 1990).

Although differences in neuropsychological outcome associated with ethnicity and other demographic variables (e.g., acculturation) have been reported in the adult HIV-1 literature (cf. Levin, Berger, Didona, & Duncan, 1992; Manly et al., 1998), the effects of such variables on performance in children with HIV-1 infection have received little attention. This is particularly the case for domains such as language and information processing speed, which are functional areas known to be highly affected by infection with this virus (cf. Brouwers et al., 1998; Cohen, Mundy, Karrassik, Lieb,

Sincere and heartfelt thanks are extended to all the children and their caretakers for their participation. The authors also extend their appreciation to Judith Rozelle for her assistance with data collection and the blind reviewers for their elucidating and constructive criticisms.

Requests for reprints should be sent to Antolin M. Llorente, Department of Pediatrics, University of Maryland School of Medicine, Mount Washington Pediatric Hospital, 1708 West Rogers Avenue, Suite 1141, Baltimore, MD 21209. E-mail: allorente@mwph.org

Ludwig, & Ward, 1991; Llorente et al., 1998; Martin et al., 1992; Wolters, Brouwers, Moss, & Pizzo, 1994).

This limitation in the neuropsychological literature is critical because both demographic (e.g., acculturation, ethnicity, socioeconomic status [SES]) and biological (e.g., genetic mutations) factors could account for differences in neuropsychological performance in HIV-infected children. With regard to demographic variables, Manly et al. (1998) demonstrated that *acculturation* (defined as the degree of assimilation and adoption of values, language, and ethnic practices of a specific culture by an individual) could account for most of the differences in performance (except for a story-learning task) between African American and European American adults with HIV-1 infection. Aside from acculturation and other demographic characteristics, biological variables are capable of accounting for ethnic-driven differences in outcome variables. In fact, HIV-1-associated central nervous system (CNS) disease in children may be influenced by genetic factors shown to play a preeminent role in disease transmission and, possibly, encephalopathy, with significant neuropsychological sequelae (cf. Sei et al., 2001). Polymorphisms in genes, particularly in chemokine receptors that affect monocytes–macrophages, have been hypothesized to affect the rate of infection or the production of cytokines by monocytes–macrophages, the main carriers of HIV-1 infection within the brain, and thus influence CNS manifestations. Such polymorphisms have been shown to resist perinatal transmission of HIV-1 in selected ethnic groups, including African American infants (cf. Kostrikis et al., 1999) and European American adults (cf. Samson et al., 1996).

This study investigated the relationship between ethnicity and neuropsychological outcome in two specific domains of functioning (language and speed of information processing) in a group of HIV-1+ children. Ethnicity in this study was defined on the basis of parental report regarding perceived ethnicity (e.g., African American, Hispanic) and primary language use (i.e., English; cf. Marin, Sabogal, Marin, Otero-Sabogal, & Perez-Stable, 1987). Because previous research has suggested that ethnicity is capable of affecting neuropsychological performance, it was postulated that differences in performance would emerge between European American children and African American children. Differences in neuropsychological performance were hypothesized to remain significant after controlling for potential confounds such as intellectual level and immunologic integrity.

Method

Participants

Twenty-two children were evaluated for this study. A large proportion of children were enrolled in antiretroviral protocols ($n = 13$; cf. Fiscus et al., 1998) as part of their participation in a comprehensive investigation examining the effects of such medications on HIV-1 infection and indirectly on the CNS. All other children were consecutively referred to a developmental clinic or pediatric hospital ($n = 9$) for a clinical neuropsychological evaluation subsequent to suspected declines in overall level of functioning ($n = 3$) or routine biannual clinical follow-up ($n = 6$). All participants were asymptomatic or mildly symptomatic HIV-1+, meeting Centers for Disease Control (CDC) criteria Category A or B (CDC, 1994). Vertically ($n = 21$; i.e., mother-to-infant) and horizontally ($n = 1$; i.e., other route of transmission) infected children were included in this study. All vertically infected children were classified as HIV-1+ if two or more cultures of peripheral blood mononuclear cells or HIV DNA were positive at any age (McIntosh et al., 1994). Horizontally infected children participating in this study had been classified as infected subsequent to positive results on two antibody tests after the age of 18 months. All children were receiving antiretroviral therapy (ART; e.g., Zidovudine [ZDV] and Dideoxyinosine [ddI] therapy).

Fifteen participants were boys, and 7 participants were girls. The average age of the participants was 6.1 ± 1.2 years at the time of assessment. All children had received an intellectual examination(s) before their participation in this investigation and overall mean with the Wechsler Intelligence Scale for Children–Third Edition (Full-Scale IQ Score [FSIQ]; Wechsler, 1991) or McCarthy Scales of Children's Abilities (General Cognitive Index [GCI]; McCarthy, 1972). Overall mean IQ standard score was 90.7 ± 2.7. English was the primary language and the language of origin for all of the children chosen for this investigation.

Materials

This investigation focused on neuropsychological correlates of HIV-1 infection on emerging one-word expressive language and information processing speed. Therefore, in addition to his or her specified antiretroviral protocol-driven neuropsychological battery in the case of children participating in a study or a battery of standardized tests in the case of children consecutively referred for clinical follow-up, each participant received procedures to assess these two domains. Emerging one-word expressive language was screened using the Expressive One-Word Picture Vocabulary Test–Revised (EOWPVT–R; Gardner, 1990), a picture-naming task. Information processing speed was screened using the Rapid Color Naming subtest from the Comprehensive Test of Phonological Processing (CTOPP; Wagner, Torgesen, & Rashotte, 1999), a Stroop-like interference test for children. Wagner et al. (1999) and Gardner (1990), respectively, reported data regarding the validity of the CTOPP and the EOWPVT–R for various healthy and clinical populations of children.

Procedure

All of the children had their diagnosis confirmed on several occasions as part of their participation in longitudinal antiretroviral studies or as part of routine medical care in the case of participants not enrolled in a research investigation. Exclusionary criteria included history of head injury or seizures, any other chronic medical condition (e.g., heart disease) except for minor opportunistic infections associated with CDC Immunologic Category B (CDC, 1994), and special education services for borderline intellectual functioning or a pervasive developmental disorder. The presence of a suspected learning disability did not disqualify participants from this study because the participants were too young to show a prominent learning disorder and because prospective participants were excluded from the study if they had been enrolled in special education classes. In addition, too few children (n = 3; 2 African American) were referred for such services after their participation in this study, precluding any type of meaningful analyses. Participants with behavioral difficulties (e.g., Attention Deficit Hyperactivity Disorder, Oppositional Defiant Disorder; n = 4) were not excluded because research has demonstrated that a large portion of behavioral problems in HIV-1-infected children are not linked to HIV disease (cf. Mellins et al., 2003). All children were afebrile at the time of their participation in this study to reduce the effect of acute illness on the results.

Although the majority of children (n = 19) had been evaluated on several occasions before their assessment for this investigation, each participant was administered the CTOPP and the EOWPVT–R only once to eliminate potential confounds, such as practice effects. The CTOPP and EOWPVT–R were administered using standardized administration procedures by qualified and trained examiners. Scoring was conducted following standard directions from each test manual. Efforts were made to assess each child before any invasive medical procedure, and the CTOPP and EOWPVT–R were always administered at the end of a research protocol or clinical test battery to avoid confounding the results from such research or clinical investigations. Intertester reliability was established and maintained through centralized training of examiners and supervisors, periodic review and clarification of scoring criteria, and selected review of assessment protocols in the case of children participating in antiretroviral research studies or established through internal procedures for children undergoing clinical follow-up. Although not consistently possible, an effort was made to keep examiners naïve to the HIV-1 infection classification category (e.g., Category B; CDC, 1994) of each child. Treatment was defined as HIV pharmacological intervention, including ZDV and other antiretroviral monotherapy (e.g., ddI) or multiantiretroviral therapy (multi-ART). Written informed consent was obtained from each participant's parent or legal guardian, and the applicable institutional review board approved all procedures. Assent was obtained from all children before their participation.

Data Analyses

Clinical, demographic, and immunologic data were analyzed using Fisher's exact probability tests. CTOPP and EOWPVT–R standard scores were analyzed separately. One-way analyses of variance using ethnic group (African American or European American) as the independent variable and CTOPP or EOWPVT–R standard scores as dependent variables were used to test differences in CTOPP and EOWPVT–R performance separately as a function of ethnicity. All statistical tests conducted during the course of this investigation were two sided, and all analyses were performed using SPSS (Version 10.0).

Results

Because clinical and immunologic variables (e.g., HIV-1 classification, CD4+ percentage) can act as potential confounds, analyses were conducted to determine whether differences in these variables emerged, thereby requiring statistical control before proceeding with analyses. Table 1 shows clinical and demographic characteristics investigated as potential confounds in this study cross-tabulated by group (African American

Table 1. *Clinical and Demographic Characteristics*[a]

	African American	European American
Children	10	12
Age: years (*SD*)	6.0 (1.4)	6.2 (1.0)
Intellect: WISC–III or MSCA Standard Score (*SD*)	90.9 (2.8)	90.5 (2.6)
ART: number/other	9/1	9/3
HIV-1 classification (CDC, 1994): number		
Class A	8	7
Class B	1	5
Missing	1	—
Maternal education: years[b]	10.2	11.9
Mean CD4+ percentage (< 29%)	8	9
Hard drug exposure in utero[c]	8	9

Note: WISC–III = Wechsler Intelligence Scale for Children–Third Edition; MSCA = McCarthy Scales for Children's Abilities; ART = antiretroviral therapy; CDC = Centers for Disease Control and Prevention.
[a]All *p* values greater than .05. [b]Used as a surrogate for socioeconomic status. [c]Crack cocaine, etc.

and European American), Group differences in these variables were not statistically significant. For this reason, in conjunction with the fact that too few participants were available to conduct meaningful and valid analyses, these variables were not used in subsequent analyses (e.g., covariates).

Table 2 shows CTOPP and EOWPVT–R standard score means and standard deviations by ethnic group. CTOPP scores differed significantly between African American and European American children, F(1, 20) = 4.86, *p* < .05, with African American children scoring lower than European American children. Similarly, EOWPVT–R scores for African American children were significantly lower than scores for European American children, *F*(1, 20) = 5.01, *p* < .05.

Discussion

Our results revealed differences in emerging one-word expressive language and information processing speed between HIV-1-infected African American and European American children. European American children performed better on both skills relative to African American children. Although not matched, the differences observed between the two groups of children in language and information processing speed reached statistical significance despite the fact that no difference in age, immunologic clinical category, intellectual ability, level of maternal education, or CD4+ percentage emerged between the two groups, as originally postulated. In addition, in an attempt to reduce the effects of other putative confounding factors capable of accounting for differences in neuropsychological outcome, children in either ethnic group were excluded from participation in this study if they met stringent and specific exclusion criteria (e.g., borderline intellectual functioning, head injury, seizures, other chronic medical conditions, or enrollment in special education services). To further reduce the potential effects of acute illness on our results, all children participating in this investigation were assessed only if they were afebrile at the time of assessment.

One explanation for these results is that African American children may have had less or limited exposure to the stimuli found in the EOWPVT–R than European American children. Although such an argument is indeed applicable to the EOWPVT–R, it is less germane to the CTOPP. This is because most children learn the colors found in this test at a very early age, and there are no pictures to name, but rather colored squares to be read as fast as possible. Alternatively, as was the case with adults (Manly et al., 1998), acculturation may have accounted for the results presented here, but because such a factor was not investigated in this study, it remains a speculative conclusion.

Table 2. *CTOPP and EOWPVT-R (Age-Corrected Standard Scores) Means and Standard Deviations as a Function of Ethnic Group*

	Ethnic Group			
	African American[a]		European American[b]	
Procedure	*M*	*SD*	*M*	*SD*
CTOPP	89.8	2.3	98.9.2	2.2
EOWPVT–R	83.5	3.2	92.7	2.3

Note: CTOPP = Comprehensive Test of Phonological Processing, Rapid Color Naming subtest; EOWPVT–R = Expressive One-Word Picture Vocabulary Test–Revised.
[a]*n* = 10. [b]*n* = 12.

The results presented here, indicative of differences in information processing speed and emerging expressive language skills between groups of African American and European American children, are consistent with previous studies conducted with HIV+ adults that examined the effects of other demographic characteristics. For example, after controlling for acculturation, most ethnic group differences disappeared in the investigation conducted by Manly et al. (1998). However, even after controlling for such a demographic variable, the results revealed that acculturation could not account for differences in performance between a group of "HIV+ African American and White" participants on a story-learning task. In other words, acculturation was incapable of accounting for all the differences in neuropsychological performance that emerged, particularly on a learning task, despite the fact that the groups were matched on "age, education, and sex." It is possible that other etiologies may account for the observed differences in performance. Biological factors, including genetic mutations, interacting with other variables (e.g., viral factors), including demographic characteristics, may partially account for the observed differences in performance. In this regard, previous research suggests that specific genetic mutations may have protective effects against HIV-1 infection, including diminishing transmission rates in select populations, including African American youth (cf. Kostrikis et al., 1999) and European American adults (Samson et al., 1996). However, some mutations also have been shown to not have significant effects on clinical outcomes (Misrahi et al., 1998) or may be modulated by other mutations, particularly those with significant CNS implications (cf. Sei et al., 2001). Therefore, in addition to acculturation, it is possible that differences in biological markers (e.g., genetic variables) interacting with other factors (e.g., virus type), including ethnicity, account for the results found in the investigation by Manly et al. and in our study; this issue merits further scrutiny. Such an interaction between biological and demographic factors also deserves special scrutiny in light of epidemiological differences found in different ethnic groups infected with HIV-1 (Hu et al., 1996; Laurent & Delaporte, 2001).

These results should be interpreted with caution and considered to be preliminary in nature, subsequent to the limitations of this investigation. Variables known to affect neurodevelopmental and neuropsychological performance in children, including birthweight, gestational age, in utero drug exposure, viral load, timing of study enrollment, and timing of infection (cf. Rodriguez et al., 1993; Smith et al., 2000), were not investigated in this study. For example, timing of infection has been shown to affect neurocognitive outcomes in children with HIV-1 infection (cf. Smith et al., 2000). Because this study did not enroll children at birth or immediately after their initial enrollment in treatment protocols, it may have failed to account for some of the early neurodevelopmental and neuropsychological manifestations associated with HIV-1 infection or treatment effects. These are issues of paramount importance, because early manifestations associated with vertical HIV-1 infection have been noted in birth cohort studies (Chase et al., 2000) and may be predictive of mortality (Llorente et al., 2003). In addition, all of these factors have been shown to be modulated by treatment.

As noted earlier, Manly et al. (1998) have shown that acculturation, even intraethnic cultural group differences, can have powerful effects on neuropsychological performance. Although probably less palpable on this young sample, this investigation unfortunately did not examine such a variable. Therefore, it is possible that level of acculturation may have affected these results. It is also possible that the definition of ethnicity used in this study failed to appropriately operationalize African American ethnicity. Such a limitation may have accounted for the differences observed in neuropsychological performance. The variable used to address SES in this investigation (maternal education) also was a rudimentary attempt to control for such a complex demographic characteristic. In that sense, it may have infringed on the accurate measurement of such a variable and indirectly on our results. Standard English language use was not formally assessed in either the children or their caretakers. Such a factor may have influenced our findings, particularly the results on the EOWPVT–R.

The fact that clinical and research subsamples were used in this investigation also may have influenced our results because differences in such subsamples may be associated with potential subject ascertainment bias such as disease severity. In addition, given that genetic data were not available, only educated conjectures can be made about the effects that such biological markers may have had, or failed to have, on our results. Pharmacological treatments, including ART therapies (multi-ART), not examined in this investigation, also may have modulated the specific neuropsychological outcomes observed in this study.

Regardless of the reason for the limitations (e.g., too few participants available to conduct meaningful and valid analyses), important relationships between ethnicity, information processing speed, and language (the domains investigated) and other areas of neuropsychological functioning and their impact on the findings presented here were not investigated. For example, because a measure of only overall intellect was available (from two different procedures with different standard deviations and indexes), potentially significant relationships between other intellectual indexes and language or information processing speed were not investigated. The intellectual index used may not have been sensitive enough to disentangle other important interactions between ethnicity and language or information processing speed. Finally, expressive language and information processing speed were narrowly defined and investigated in this study. Broader assessments of these domains may provide different results.

Despite the caveats noted here, these findings are promising and have significant applied implications. These results buttress the need for careful assessments of children with HIV-1 from ethnic minority backgrounds, considering the effect of ethnicity on test result interpretation. As noted by Manly et al. (1998), our results also argue in favor of developing separate "ethnic group norms" for African Americans (including children) that would lead to improved diagnostic and neuropsychological performance delineation over demographically corrected norms currently available, which include normative samples predominantly based on European American cohorts. With regard to research, these results warrant further investigation. Future studies should investigate the effect of acculturation on neuropsychological performance in HIV+ African American children and other pediatric ethnic groups relative to European American children. Similarly, future studies should examine the role of genetic mutations in infected African American youth to determine whether such mutations can have beneficial effects on neurodevelopmental and neuropsychological outcomes, as has been found for other clinical outcomes (e.g., disease transmission, progression; cf. Kostrikis et al., 1999). Studies using large birth cohorts of children from various ethnic backgrounds also should be conducted while controlling for potential confounds not examined in this study to determine the effects of such variables on neuropsychological performance. Finally, the study of the relationships between treatment, particularly recent pharmacological interventions (e.g., HAART), ethnicity, and neuropsychological outcomes, deserves further attention.

References

Belman, A. L., Ultmann, M. H., Horoupian, D., et al. (1985). Neurological complications in infants and children with acquired immune deficiency syndrome. *Annals of Neurology, 18,* 560–566.

Brouwers, P., Wolters, P., & Civitello, L. (1998). Central nervous system manifestations and assessment. In P. A. Pizzo & C. M. Wilfert (Eds.), *Pediatric AIDS: The challenge of HIV infection in infants, children, and adolescents* (3rd ed., pp. 293–308). Baltimore: Williams & Wilkins.

Centers for Disease Control and Prevention. (1994). Centers for Disease Control and Prevention: 1994 revised classification system for human immunodeficiency virus infection in children less than 13 years of age. *Morbidity and Mortality Weekly Report, 43,* 1.

Chase, C., Ware, J., Hittleman, J., et al. (2000). Early cognitive and motor development among infants born to women infected by human immunodeficiency virus. *Pediatrics, 106,* 25.

Cohen, S., Mundy, T., Karrassik, B., Lieb, L., Ludwig, D., & Ward, J. (1991). Neuropsychological functioning in human immunodeficiency virus type 1 seropositive children infected through neonatal blood transfusion. *Pediatrics, 88,* 58–68.

Ellis, R. J., Deutsch, R., Heaton, R. K., et al. (1997). Neurocognitive impairment is an independent risk factor for death in HIV infection. *Archives of Neurology, 54,* 416–424.

Epstein, L. G., Sharer, L. R., Joshi, V. V., Fojas, M. M., Koenigsberger, M. R., & Oleske, J. M. (1985). Progressive encephalopathy in children with acquired immune deficiency syndrome. *Annals of Neurology, 17,* 488–496.

Fiscus, S. A., Hughes, M. D., Lathey, J. L., et al. (1998). Changes in virologic markers as predictors of CD4 cell decline and progression of disease in human immunodeficiency virus type 1-infected adults treated with nucleosides. AIDS Clinical Trials Group Protocol 175 Team. *Journal of Infectious Diseases, 177,* 625–633.

Gardner, M. F. (1990). *Expressive One-Word Picture Vocabulary Test–Revised manual.* Novato, CA: Academic Therapy Publications.

Hu, D. J., Dondero, T. J., Rayfield, M. A., et al. (1996). The emerging genetic diversity of HIV. The importance of global surveillance for diagnostics, research, and prevention. *Journal of the American Medical Association, 275,* 210–216.

Kostrikis, L. G., Neumann, A. V., Thomson, B., et al. (1999). A polymorphism in the regulatory region of the CC-Chemokine Receptor 5 gene influences perinatal transmission of human immunodeficiency virus type-1 to African-American infants. *Journal of Virology, 73,* 10264–10271.

Laurent, C., & Delaporte, E. (2001). Epidemiology of HIV infection in sub-Saharan Africa. *AIDS Review, 3,* 59–66.

Levin, B. E., Berger, J. R., Didona, T., & Duncan, R. (1992). Cognitive function in asymptomatic HIV-1 infection: The effects of age, education, ethnicity, and depression. *Neuropsychology, 6,* 303–313.

Llorente, A. M., Brouwers, P., Charurat, M., et al. (2003). Early neurodevelopmental markers predictive of mortality in infants infected with HIV-1. *Developmental Medicine and Child Neurology, 45,* 76–84.

Llorente, A. M., LoPresti, C. M., & Satz, P. (1997). Neuropsychological and neurobehavioral sequelae associated with pediatric HIV infection. In C. R. Reynolds & E. Fletcher-Janzen (Eds.), *Handbook of clinical child neuropsychology* (2nd ed., pp. 634–650). New York: Plenum.

Llorente, A. M., Miller, E. N., D'Elia, L. F., et al. (1998). Slowed information processing in HIV-1 disease. The Multicenter AIDS

Cohort Study (MACS). *Journal of Clinical and Experimental Neuropsychology, 20,* 60–72.

Lyman, W. D., Kress, Y., Kure, K., Rashbaum, W. K., Rubinstein, A., & Seira, R. (1990). Detection of HIV in fetal central nervous system tissue. *AIDS, 4,* 917–920.

Manly, J. L., Miller, S. W., Heaton, R. K., et al. (1998). The effect of African-American acculturation on neuropsychological test performance in normal and HIV-positive individuals. The HIV Neurobehavioral Research Center (HNRC) Group. *Journal of the International Neuropsychological Society, 4,* 291–302.

Marin, G., Sabogal, F., Marin, B. V. B., Otero-Sabogal, R., & Perez-Stable, E. J. (1987). Development of a short acculturation scale for Hispanics. *Hispanic Journal of Behavioral Sciences, 9,* 182–205.

Martin, E. M., Robertson, L. C., Edelstein, H. E., et al. (1992). Performance of patients with early HIV-1 infection on the Stroop Task. *Journal of Clinical and Experimental Neuropsychology, 14,* 857–868.

McCarthy, D. (1972). *Manual for the McCarthy Scales of Children's Abilities.* New York: Psychological Corporation.

McIntosh, K., Pitt, J., Banbrilla, D., et al. (1994). Blood culture in the first 6 months of life in for the diagnosis of vertically transmitted human immunodeficiency virus infection. *Journal of Infectious Diseases, 170,* 996–1000.

Mellins, C. A., Smith, R., O'Driscoll, P., et al. (2003). High rates of behavioral problems in perinatally HIV-infected children are not linked to HIV disease. *Pediatrics, 111,* 384–393.

Misrahi, M., Teglas, J.-P., N'Go, N., et al. (1998). CCR5 chemokine receptor variant in HIV-1 mother-to-child transmission and disease progression in children. *Journal of the American Medical Association , 279,* 277–280.

Rodriguez, E. M., Mendez, H., Rich, K., et al. (1993). Maternal drug use in perinatal HIV studies: The Women and Infants Transmission Study. *Annals of the New York Academy of Sciences, 693,* 245–248.

Samson, M., Libert, F., Doranz, B. J., et al. (1996). Resistance to HIV-1 infection in European-American individuals bearing mutant alleles of the CCR5 chemokine receptor gene. *Nature, 382,* 722–725.

Sei, S., Boler, A. M., Nguyen, G. T., et al. (2001). Protective effect of CCR5 delta 32 heterozygosity is restricted by SDF-1 genotype in children with HIV-1 infection. *AIDS, 15,* 1343–1352.

Sharer, L. R., Dowling, P., Micheals, J., & Cook, S. D. (1990). Spinal cord disease in children with HIV-1 infection: A combined biological and neuropathological study. *Neuropathology and Applied Neurobiology, 16,* 317–331.

Smith, R., Malee, K., Charurat, M., et al. (2000). Timing of perinatal human immunodeficiency virus type-1 infection and rate of neurodevelopment. The Women and Infant Transmission Study Group. *Pediatric Infectious Disease Journal, 19,* 862–871.

Wagner, R. K., Torgesen, J. K., & Rashotte, C. A. (1999). *The Comprehensive Test of Phonological Processing: Examiner's manual.* Austin, TX: PRO-ED.

Wechsler, D. (1991). *Wechsler Intelligence Scale for Children–Third Edition.* San Antonio, TX: Psychological Corporation.

Wolters, P., Brouwers, P., Moss, H., & Pizzo, P. (1994). Adaptive behavior of children with symptomatic HIV infection before and after Zidovudine therapy. *Journal of Pediatric Psychology, 19,* 47–61.

Applied Neuropsychology
2004, Vol. 11, No. 1, 54–64

Perception of Health and Quality of Life in Minorities After Mild-to-Moderate Traumatic Brain Injury

Sharon A. Brown

Department of Physical Medicine and Rehabilitation, and Department of Psychiatry and Behavioral Sciences, Baylor College of Medicine, Houston, Texas, USA

Stephen R. McCauley

Department of Physical Medicine and Rehabilitation, Baylor College of Medicine, Houston, Texas, USA

Harvey S. Levin

Department of Physical Medicine and Rehabilitation, Department of Psychiatry and Behavioral Sciences, and Department of Neurosurgery, Baylor College of Medicine, Houston, Texas, USA

Charles Contant

Department of Neurosurgery, Baylor College of Medicine, Houston, Texas, USA

Corwin Boake

University of Texas Health Science Center, Houston, Texas, USA

Much has been reported of the influence of age, affective symptoms, and satisfaction on self-ratings of health functioning, but little is known about the extent that race-based perceptions may have on influencing behavior or adjustment after a mild-to-moderate traumatic brain injury (MTBI). We investigated differences in perception of health functioning by race for mental and physical functioning using a global measure of health functioning. MTBI (n = 135) and general trauma (GT, n = 83) patients recruited from an area Level-1 trauma center at 3 months after injury were administered the Medical Outcomes Study: Short Form (SF-36), Structured Clinical Interview for the Diagnostic and Statistical Manual of Mental Disorders (4th ed.; American Psychiatric Association, 1994), Community Integration Questionnaire, Social Support Questionnaire (SSQ), Center for Epidemiological Studies–Depression, and the Visual Analogue Scale of Depression. A significant interaction for Race × Group (p < .01) was found on the Physical Component Scale (PCS) of the SF-36. In the MTBI group, African Americans reported worse functioning (p < .04) on the PCS scale; they perceived functioning on subscales General Health Perception (p < .02) and Physical Functioning (p < .04) to be more limited. On the SSQ, Hispanic MTBI patients reported having fewer social supports available to them (p < .05), although the race groups were comparable for satisfaction with their support. Rate of depression across groups was comparable, although subjective reporting by minority MTBI patients indicated greater depressed feelings. Differences in perception of health functioning may be related to the unique interaction created between sustaining an MTBI and variations in cultural expression of disability. Manifestations of physical difficulties may be better accepted for some cultures than having mental illness.

Key words: mild traumatic brain injury, health perception, depression, ethnic minority

This research was supported by the CDC, Grant No. R49/CCR 612707.

Requests for reprints should be sent to Sharon A. Brown, Cognitive Neuroscience Laboratory, Baylor College of Medicine, Department of Psychiatry and Behavioral Science and Physical Medicine and Rehabilitation, 6560 Fannin, Ste. 1144, Box 67, Houston, TX 77030. E-mail: sbrown@bcm.tmc.edu

There currently is a void in the understanding of how cultural or ethnic differences relate to the recovery process and what factors are relevant to enhancing recovery. The influence of age, ethnicity, affective symptoms, and satisfaction affect self-ratings of general health functioning, yet little is known of the extent to which different cultural conceptions of traumatic brain injury (TBI) are negative or stigmatizing and how such stigma may influence patterns of behavior and adjustment (Simpson, Mohr, & Redman, 2000). Within the TBI literature, few studies have examined functional outcome as a function of ethnicity. Of those that have, differences were not significant for either functional outcome and community integration or level of cognition and functional outcome at admission and discharge between minorities and European Americans in patients with mild TBI (Burnett, Silver, Kolakowsky-Hayner, & Cifu, 2000; Rosenthal et al., 1996).

Ascertaining perception of health functioning or adjustment to disability after TBI has become an important indicator of functional outcome. The Medical Outcomes Study: Short Form-36 (SF-36) is one of the most widely used measures for assessing quality of health (Ware & Sherbourne, 1992). Its use in TBI research is increasing, and it has been demonstrated to be sensitive to short- and longer term outcomes after TBI and to be a reliable and valid measure for assessing health functioning after TBI (Bullinger et al., 2002; Corrigan, Smith-Knapp, & Granger, 1998; Findler, Cantor, Haddad, Gordon, & Ashman, 2001; Paniak, Phillips, Toller-Lobe, Durand, & Nagy, 1999). The SF-36 is able to assess non-TBI issues, such as bodily pain and the functional effects of musculoskeletal injuries, which can be important in predicting outcomes after mild TBI (Dacey, Dikmen, Temkin, McLean, Armsden, & Winn, 1991; Paniak et al., 1999). The SF-36 mental, physical, and general health subscales were sensitive to the effects of posttraumatic stress disorder in trauma patients (71% of whom sustained blunt trauma), and the role-functioning subscale was sensitive to the effects of depression or anxiety in mild TBI patients (Fann, Katon, Vomoto, & Esselman, 1995; Michaels, Michaels, Smith, Moon, Peterson, & Long, 2000). During the acute stages of recovery, the SF-36 demonstrated significance in detecting perceptions of functioning between mild TBI patients and control participants (Paniak et al., 1999). Over time, the SF-36 measures were used to track improvement from 6 to 12 months after injury and detected areas of least improvement in functioning in trauma patients (Michaels et al., 2000).

Studies to date on the assessment of health functioning after TBI are limited, and the results are mixed, depending on the question asked. Some investigators report that comorbidities, including orthopedic injuries and mood disorders, contribute to lowered self-ratings of health functioning (Fann et al., 1995; Michaels et al., 1999). This study represents preliminary work investigating racial differences in perception of health functioning after TBI. Specifically, we asked, do African American and Hispanic American patients rate their health as poor relative to European Americans, and what other factors contribute to lowered ratings? Are there differences in emotional functioning along ethnic divisions that contribute to general health functioning?

Method

Participants

Patients with mild-to-moderate TBI (MTBI) and patients sustaining general trauma (GT) were recruited from Ben Taub General Hospital, a Level-1 trauma center affiliated with Baylor College of Medicine. *Mild TBI* was defined as a closed head injury producing a period of unconsciousness of no longer than 20 min, lowest postresuscitation score of 13–15 on the Glasgow Coma Scale (GCS) of Teasdale and Jennett (1974), no extracranial injury that necessitated surgical repair under general anesthesia, and computed tomographic (CT) findings within 24 hr after injury indicating normal intracranial findings or a brain lesion that did not require surgical evacuation. A TBI was classified as *moderate* if the lowest postresuscitation GCS score was 9–12 with or without evidence of lesion on CT. Inclusion criteria included residence within Harris County and an age range of 16 years or older. Bilingual examiners obtained consent and administered assessments to monolingual Spanish-speaking participants. Exclusion criteria included penetrating missile injury of the brain, a history of diagnosed schizophrenia, mental deficiency, hospitalization for previous TBI, history of treatment for recent substance abuse, and a blood alcohol level exceeding 200 mg/dL when examined in the emergency center (EC). To control for risk factors predisposing to traumatic injury, a comparison group of adults who were treated after sustaining extracranial traumatic injury was recruited during the same period as the TBI patients. Extracranial injury severity in the TBI and GT groups was measured using the Injury Severity Score (ISS; Baker, O'Neill, Haddon, & Long, 1974). The ISS is the sum of the squares of the highest Abbreviated Injury Scale score in each of the three most severely injured body regions (head and neck, face, chest, abdominal or pelvic contents, extremities, and external). The ISS was modified to represent the three most severely injured body areas, excluding the head. Before discharge from the EC or hospital, demographic information and informed consent were obtained from all patients.

Procedures

Outpatient evaluations were scheduled at 3 months (± 2 weeks) and 6 months (± 1 month) after injury to assess emotional and cognitive functioning and functional outcome. Given the attrition rates between 3 and 6 months after injury and previous studies indicating that the 3-month interval was sufficient to identify and study the neurobehavioral sequelae of MTBI, this article reports the 3-month data (Dikmen, McLean, & Temkin, 1986; Fenton, McClelland, Montgomery, MacFlynn, & Rutherford, 1993; Levin et al., 1987; Ponsford et al., 2000; Rimel, Giordani, Barth, & Jane, 1982).

Health Perception

The SF-36 was given as a measure of the patient's perception of health status for physical and mental functioning (Ware & Sherbourne, 1992). The SF-36 permits scoring of a set of eight scales displayed as a profile of health status concepts. The items and scales were constructed for scoring using the Likert method of summated ratings. The raw scores are transformed to scaled scores (i.e., percentages) ranging from 0–100, in which higher scores reflected better perceived health or less impact of health problems on functioning. The Mental Component Summary (MCS) score and Physical Component Scale (PCS) score are two standardized composite scores that summarize the eight domain scores. Higher scores reflect better functioning. The summary scales and index scales served as dependent variables.

Functional Outcome

The Community Integration Questionnaire (CIQ) was given to measure resumption of roles in family, community, and social domains (Willer, Rosenthal, Kreutzer, Gordon, & Rempel, 1993). All domains and the total score (summation across domains) were used as the measures of interest. Lower scores reflected poorer functioning. The Social Support Questionnaire (SSQ) provided a measure of the number of persons available for support and satisfaction with the available support system (Sarason, Sarason, & Shearin, 1987). Higher scores indicated more support and better satisfaction.

Mood Functioning

The primary measure of depression was the nonpatient version of the Structured Clinical Interview (SCID) for the *Diagnostic and Statistical Manual of Mental Disorders* (4th ed.; *DSM-IV*; American Psychiatric Association, 1994), a form designed for studies of populations without a known diagnosis of depression (First, Spitzer, Gibbon, & Williams, 1995). Based on the SCID, the research technician and a supervising psychologist determined whether the patient met *DSM-IV* criteria for diagnosis of major depressive episode (MDE) either during the first 3 months after injury or at any point in his or her lifetime before the injury. The interview was audiotaped and reviewed by one of the authors of the SCID as a check for consistency in measurement administration and scoring.

The Center for Epidemiological Studies–Depression (CES–D) and the Visual Analogue Scale of Depression (VASD) were used as a measure of severity of depressive symptomatology (Aitken, 1969; Radloff, 1977). The CES–D, a 20-item self-report questionnaire, asked respondents to rate their depressive symptoms during the past week on a 5-point Likert scale ranging from 0 (*none of the time*) to 3 (*all of the time*). The CES–D has fewer somatic items than other widely used scales of depression and has been used in epidemiological studies of depression (Boyd, Weissman, Thompson, & Myers, 1982). The VASD asked patients to typify their current mood by placing a mark on a 100-mm horizontal line between endpoints of "I am not depressed" to "I have never been more depressed." The total CES–D score and the distance in millimeters from the nondepressed endpoint to the participant's mark on the VASD were used as the dependent measures.

Design and Statistical Analyses

All data analyses were carried out with Statistical Analysis Software for Windows Version 8.2. *Statistical significance* was defined as $p < .05$ for all analyses, unless otherwise stated. Nonparametric statistics were used for measures that were not normally distributed. Fisher's exact probability test was used instead of chi-square when proportions were markedly unbalanced (more extreme than 80%/20%) or when at least one cell size was less than 5.

Results

Patient accrual from August 1999 to March 2001 included 399 patients sustaining MTBI and 255 sustaining GT. Of these, 264 MTBI patients and 172 GT trauma patients were lost to follow-up. Comparison of patients lost to follow-up and those retained revealed significant differences for demographic indexes. The modal patient lost to follow-up was less educated, Hispanic American, monolingual Spanish speaking, and sustained injury as a result of an assault (Table 1). A description of the demographic information of the MTBI and GT patients who were eligible for the 3-month evaluation is provided in Table 2. The proportion of minority patients in the MTBI group was comparable with that within the GT group. The MTBI and GT groups also were comparable for age, education, occupation, and injury severity (using the ISS). The groups differed by mechanism of injury (Fisher's exact probability, $p <$ .008). Twice the number of MTBI patients were injured as a result of a motor vehicle accident or assault compared with GT patients.

Table 1. *Demographic and Injury Characteristics of Patients Retained and Lost to Follow-Up*

	Retained		Lost to Follow-Up		
	M	SD	M	SD	p
Ethnicity					.01
European American	45		85		
Hispanic American	109		264		
African American	64		87		
Gender	61 F/157 M		100 F/336 M		.03
Age	34.28	13.85	32.22	12.48	.06
Education	11.16	3.21	9.93	3.60	< .001
GCS-EC	14.67	1.12	14.69	1.10	< .79
Pre-IQ	96.72	7.02	94.14	70.06	< .001
ISS	4.05	5.38	3.51	5.70	.24
Occupation					.02
Language (English/Spanish)	154/61		250/181		.0007
Mechanism of injury					.006
Assault	32		105		
Fall	27		54		
MVA	151		247		
Other	8		30		

Note: GCS-EC = Glasgow Coma Scale-Emergency Center; ISS = injury severity score; MVA = motor vehicle accident.

Table 2. *Demographic and Injury Characteristics of MTBI and GT Patients*

	MTBI		GT		
	M	SD	M	SD	p
Ethnicity					.35
European American	28		17		
Hispanic American	63		46		
African American	44		20		
Gender	37 F/98 M		24 F/59 M		.81
Age	33.94	14.52	34.85	12.73	.64
Education	11.07	3.48	11.31	2.70	.59
GCS-EC	14.47	1.38	15.00	0.00	< .001
Pre-IQ	9.57	7.02	96.96	7.06	.69
ISS	4.28	5.90	3.67	4.40	.41
Occupation					.28
Mechanism of injury					.01
Assault	22		10		
Fall	10		17		
MVA	100		51		
Other	3		5		

Note: MTBI = mild-to-moderate traumatic brain injury; GT = general trauma; GCS-EC = Glasgow Coma Scale-Emergency Center; ISS = injury severity score; MVA = motor vehicle accident.

Table 3. *Medical Outcomes Study: Short Form PCS and MCS Scale Performance for MTBI and GT Patients*

	MTBI[a]		GT[b]	
	M	*SD*	*M*	*SD*
PCS	44.98	9.79	42.21	11.47
Physical functioning	74.23	26.91	67.41	29.10
Role—physical	47.78	41.03	36.75	41.38
Pain index	58.43	25.71	59.58	28.32
General health perception	63.07	22.49	65.89	24.46
MCS	41.45	13.29	44.74	13.69
Vitality	53.56	21.92	55.54	26.07
Social functioning	65.37	27.82	65.96	26.07
Role—emotional	48.15	42.84	52.21	42.67
Mental health index	59.33	24.75	64.65	26.16

Note: PCS = Physical Component Scale; MCS = Mental Component Scale; MTBI = mild-to-moderate traumatic brain injury; GT = general trauma.
[a]$n = 135$. [b]$n = 80$.

Mental and Physical Health Perception

The MCS and PCS scales of the SF-36 were analyzed to measure the patient's perception of his or her health functioning. No significant differences were noted for the MCS scale (Table 3, Figure 1) or any of its subscales by ethnicity. However, on the PCS scale, a significant two-way interaction, $F(5, 212) = 3.05$ $p < .01$, was found for Group × Ethnicity.

PCS and Injury Group

To better understand the Group × Ethnicity interaction, analyses were conducted to examine patient group differences. Comparison between the MTBI group and the GT group on the PCS scale did not reveal a main effect for group, although a trend was indicated, $F(1, 216) = 3.60$, $p = .059$. Individual subscale differences were explored. Of the four subscales, only the Role Physical Index, Kruskal–Wallis $\chi^2(1, N = 216) = 3.78$, $p = .05$, was able to detect a trend for group difference. Patients in the GT group reported experiencing greater limitations in ability to perform physical activities related to work, self-care, and social activities, relative to patients in the MTBI group.

PCS and Ethnicity

Further analysis of the Group × Ethnicity interaction revealed a significant main effect for ethnicity, $F(2,$

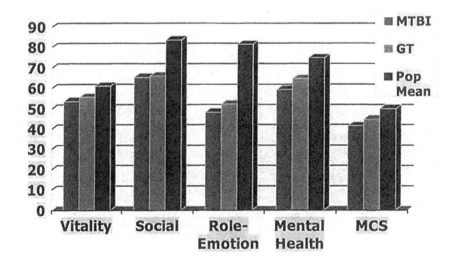

Figure 1. Medical Outcomes Study: Short Form Mental Component Scale scores for the MTBI and GT groups. Higher scores indicate better functioning. MTBI = mild-to-moderate brain injury; GT = general trauma; Pop Mean = SF–36 Population Mean Score; MCS = Mental Component Summary.

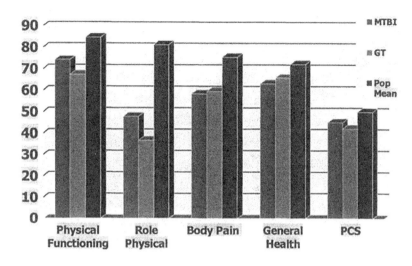

Figure 2. Medical Outcomes Study: Short Form Physical Component Scale scores for the MTBI and GT groups. Higher scores indicate better functioning. MTBI = mild-to-moderate brain injury; GT = general trauma; Pop Mean = SF–36 Population Mean Score; PCS = Physical Component Scale.

215) = 3.78, $p < .02$. Within-patient group differences were then compared. Within the MTBI group, the PCS scale differed significantly by ethnicity, $F(2, 132) = 3.31, p < .04$. African Americans reported worse functioning than Hispanic Americans, who, in turn, reported that their overall level of functioning was at a level comparable to European Americans (Table 4). The subscales of the PCS were then analyzed. Two indexes were significant: the General Health Perception Index, Kruskal–Wallis $\chi^2(2, N = 131) = 8.05, p < .02$, and the Physical Functioning Index, Kruskal–Wallis $\chi^2(2, N = 131) = 6.46, p < .04$. As can be seen in Figure 3, on the General Health Index, African Americans rated their health functioning to be poor relative to European Americans and Hispanic Americans, who were not significantly different from one another. On the Physical Functioning Index scale, African Americans perceived their ability to perform physical activities, which included bathing or dressing (activities of daily living), as more limited than Hispanic Americans or European Americans. It is interesting to note that Hispanic Americans reported a relatively high level of performance in physical functioning. Although not statistically significant, African Americans reported experiencing greater levels of pain than European Americans or Hispanic Americans.

Differences found were not readily attributable to differences related to demographics. Analysis of the demographic information of the MTBI group by ethnicity revealed no significant differences for age, GCS score obtained at admission to the EC, mechanism of injury, gender, injury severity, and occupation. However, the groups differed significantly for years of education, $F(2, 132) = 11.76, p = .0001$. Hispanic American MTBI patients completed fewer formal years of education ($M = 9.7$ years, $SD = 3.74$) relative to European Americans ($M = 13.0$ years, $SD = 2.85$) and African Americans ($M = 11.8$ years, $SD = 2.61$).

Table 4. *MTBI Group Racial Differences on the Medical Outcomes Study: Short Form*

	European American[a]		Hispanic American[b]		African American[c]	
	M	*SD*	*M*	*SD*	*M*	*SD*
Physical Component Scale*	46.01	10.35	46.64	8.69	41.93	10.41
Physical functioning	75.71	25.19	80.31	23.08	64.60	30.66
Role—physical*	51.79	42.99	49.21	41.87	43.18	39.02
Pain index	60.61	25.87	62.16	24.23	51.70	26.90
General health perception	68.43	21.59	66.44	23.11	55.95	20.80

Note: MTBI = mild-to-moderate traumatic brain injury.
[a]$n = 28.$ [b]$n = 63.$ [c]$n = 44.$
*$p < .05.$

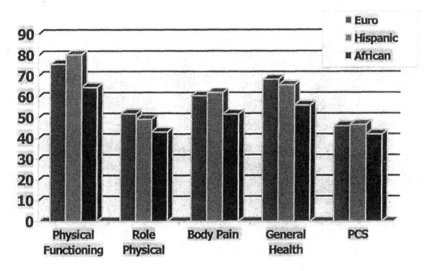

Figure 3. Medical Outcomes Study: Short Form Physical Component Scale scores by ethnicity for the MTBI group. Higher scores indicate better functioning. PCS = Physical Component Scale.

Functional Outcome

Functional outcome was assessed to determine its contribution to perception of functioning. The SSQ provided an indication of currently available social network. The CIQ provided a measure of resumption of previous life roles.

Group Difference for SSQ and CIQ

A significant two-way interaction, $F(5, 211) = 4.07$, $p < .001$, was detected (Group × Ethnicity) for the number of persons available for support (Social Support Questionnaire Number of Supports [SSQNS]). To better understand the interaction effect, further analyses were conducted examining effect of group and ethnicity on the SSQNS. A main effect was detected for ethnicity, $F(2, 214) = 3.12$, $p < .05$, and more specifically between Hispanic American patients ($M = 2.37$ support persons) and European American participants ($M = 3.19$ support persons; Table 5). Comparisons were then made examining ethnic differences within patient group. Within the GT group, a significant difference, $F(2, 79) = 5.31$, $p < .007$, was noted between African Americans and Hispanic Americans and between Euro-

pean Americans and Hispanic Americans (Table 5). African Americans tended to have more persons available for support relative to European Americans, who, in turn, reported more support persons available than Hispanic Americans.

Evaluation of Mood

Analyses were conducted to investigate the contribution of mood functioning. The CES-D and VASD measured degree of depressive symptom severity and subjective perception of how depressed patients felt, respectively. Although rates of depression, based on SCID ratings, were comparable between groups, scores on the VASD revealed a significant Group × Ethnicity interaction, $F(5, 211) = 2.49$, $p < .03$. Analyses were performed assessing main effects for group. A main effect for patient group, $F(1, 215) = 7.39$, $p < .007$, was detected. That is, patients in the MTBI group reported feeling more depressed (M VASD score = 39.45, $SD = 34.84$) than those in the GT group (M VASD score = 26.66, $SD = 31.68$).

Several areas failed to demonstrate significance. Within the GT group, no main effect of ethnicity was

Table 5. *Number of Support Persons Available by Ethnicity*

	European American		Hispanic American		African American		
SSQNS Groups	M	SD	M	SD	M	SD	p
GT and MTBI[a]	3.19	1.98	2.37	1.67	2.59	2.03	.04
GT[b]	3.59	2.26	2.11	1.85	3.69	2.55	.007
MTBI[c]	2.94	1.79	2.55	1.51	2.09	1.53	.08

Note: SSQNS = Social Support Questionnaire Number of Supports; GT = general trauma; MTBI = mild-to-moderate traumatic brain injury.
[a]$n = 218$. [b]$n = 83$. [c]$n = 135$.

detected on the PCS scale and the subscales that constitute it. When ethnicity was held constant across the PCS scale, no effect was found between the MTBI and GT patient groups. On the SSQ, patient group main effects were not demonstrated for number of supports available. Within the MTBI group, ethnic differences were not demonstrated on the SSQNS. Satisfaction (SSQSS) with available support network demonstrated no group differences. Scores on the CIQ and its subscales (home, social, productivity, and total) failed to demonstrate any group differences within or between patient and ethnic groups. Assessment of mood revealed no significant group differences based on the CES-D scores, although African Americans had higher rates of symptom severity in both the MTBI and GT groups (Table 6). No main effect for ethnicity was found on the VASD, although African Americans tended to report greater subjective feelings of depression in the MTBI group.

Discussion

By assessing functional outcome after TBI, clinicians are provided with a measure of the extent of recovery or resumption of premorbid levels of activity. After an MTBI, recovery of function generally occurs within the first 3 months after injury. However, when the patient's perception of his or her health functioning is obtained, results suggest that not all patients report their functioning has fully returned to the preinjury level. Our findings suggest that ethnicity may play a significant role in the patient's perception of his or her current level of health functioning. We compared a sample of patients sustaining MTBI to a group of patients who sustained GT who were comparable for injury severity (excluding the head) and other (demographic) risk factors associated with TBI. We found a significant interaction for ethnicity and injury. Specifically, minority MTBI patients reported having significantly worse health, particularly for physical functioning relative to patients who sustained GT.

The SF-36 was used to ascertain patient perception of health functioning. MTBI and GT patients reported similar levels of functioning when asked to rate their current health; mental and physical health ratings were comparable, although the ratings were lower than the normative sample of the SF-36. Our findings were similar to those of Deane, Pigott, and Dearing (1996), who found no significant differences between MTBI patients and control participants using the General Health Perceptions Index to assess health perception. Counter to the findings in this study, Paniak et al. (1999) found worse functioning reported by MTBI patients relative to control participants assessed at 3 weeks using the SF-36. Dikmen et al. (1986), however, used the Sickness Impact Profile at 1 month after injury and found results similar to Paniak's group of MTBI patients reporting significant dysfunction for physically related activities (e.g., ambulation, body care, and movement) relative to uninjured control participants. Orthopedic-related injuries were asserted to contribute to the ratings of worse health functioning. This finding might be anticipated, given that the patients were in the early stages of recovery from injury. An ad-

Table 6. *Mood Functioning in the MTBI and GT Patient Groups*

Group	European American		Hispanic American		African American		
	M	SD	M	SD	M	SD	p
TBI[a]							
CESD	17.89	15.98	21.62	14.28	24.91	13.93	.14
VASD	32.41	35.74	37.02	32.79	47.25	36.48	.16
CIQ-home	6.04	3.07	5.33	2.87	4.68	3.26	.18
CIQ-social	5.43	2.46	6.38	2.19	5.55	2.29	.08
CIQ-productive	4.57	1.60	4.79	2.06	4.59	1.83	.28
CIQ-total	16.36	4.51	16.52	4.59	14.82	3.80	.12
GT[b]							
CESD	17.53	13.93	18.89	14.88	19.65	14.24	.90
VASD	21.18	28.05	30.09	33.25	23.45	31.35	.53
CIQ-home	6.50	2.88	5.76	3.49	5.40	3.02	.63
CIQ-social	5.86	3.01	6.16	1.85	5.95	1.76	.87
CIQ-productive	4.71	2.05	4.40	2.00	4.65	2.01	.80
CIQ-total	18.36	5.08	16.58	3.96	16.00	4.07	.26

Note: MTBI = mild-to-moderate traumatic brain injury; GT = general trauma; CESD = Center for Epidemiological Studies–Depression; VASD = Visual Analogue Scale of Depression; CIQ = Community Integration Questionnaire.
[a]n = 135. [b]n = 83.

vantage of assessing patients at 3 months after injury and using a comparison group of GT patients recruited simultaneously helped differentiate the effects attributable solely to orthopedic injuries or other nonspecific effects of sustaining a traumatic injury.

Our study noted a trend for the GT group members to view their physical functioning as more limited relative to the MTBI group; however, this trend did not fully explain the interaction. Given that the groups were comparable for injury severity and demographics, within-group differences were thought to better account for the effect. As such, we examined differences for ethnicity within patient group. Within the MTBI group, African Americans reported having the worst health functioning, whereas Hispanic Americans and European Americans reported similar levels of functioning. African Americans consistently reported lower levels of functioning across all subscales of the PCS, with significantly worse functioning noted for performing physical activities of daily living (e.g., dressing and bathing) and for general health functioning. This finding was similar to the findings of others, showing lowered ratings for physical functioning by African Americans with other medical conditions. Data reported from the national survey of families and households assessing global health and functional limitations of daily living in a sample of more than 12,000 found that the percentage of African Americans reporting increased functional limitations of daily activities was significantly greater than the percentage of European Americans (Ren & Amick, 1996). Jackson-Triche and others (Jackson-Triche, Greer Sullivan, Wells, Rogers, Camp, & Mazel, 2000) found that African Americans reported having the poorest quality of life in their study examining health-related quality of life. Linn, Hunter, and Linn (1980) found highest rating of disability among African Americans for activities of daily living in their sample of elderly patients presenting to the ambulatory care clinic at a university medical center. Unique to our study was the finding that Hispanic American patients had better ratings of health functioning for physical activity, whereas others have shown poorer ratings by persons of Hispanic descent. Linn et al. found the self-report of elderly Cubans was rated as significantly more limited. More Hispanic Americans rated their global health as poorest relative to European Americans and second to African Americans (Ren & Amick, 1996). Shetterly, Baxter, Mason, and Hamman (1996) found Hispanic American diabetic patients were three times more likely to report their health as poor or fair rather than good or excellent relative to non-Hispanic Whites.

We found a tendency for African Americans to report relatively greater levels of pain, similar to the findings by Linn et al. of higher levels of pain experienced by African Americans reported, even when level of impairment did not differ significantly by culture.

Differences in perception of functioning did not appear to result directly from injury-related or demographic measures, as there were no significant differences for ethnicity on these measures, with the exception of years of education. Hispanic American patients had fewer years of formal education, whereas African Americans and European Americans completed similar numbers of years of schooling. Other factors thought to potentially contribute to ethnic differences included the possibility of a mood disorder and functional outcome. Although depression has been reported to be strongly related to subjective ratings of quality of life and has accounted for a significant amount of variance in TBI patients, we did not find significant effects for rates of depression and severity of depressive symptoms by patient group or by ethnicity (Brown, Gordon, & Haddad, 2000; Granger, Divan, & Fiedler, 1995). However, subjective rating of depressive symptoms was greater in MTBI patients, with a tendency noted for African Americans to report feeling more depressed than European Americans and Hispanic Americans. The proportion of African Americans (18%) meeting diagnostic criteria for an MDE tended to be only slightly higher than that of European Americans (11%) and Hispanic Americans (17%). Jackson-Triche et al. (2000) also noted rates of depressive symptoms to be highest among African Americans and Hispanic Americans. Functional outcome, as measured by resumption of previous role activities, did not contribute to our understanding of perception of functioning in MTBI patents. Having several persons available for social support, however, was of significance, and Hispanic Americans reported having more persons available. This effect, however, did not hold true within the MTBI patient group.

A possible explanation for the interaction between MTBI and ethnicity would be the unique situation created between the sequelae associated with a brain injury and its interaction with cultural variations. Personality and cultural variables are asserted to influence MTBI patients' perceptions about their disability (Prigatano, 1999) and thereby affect or influence response to specific questions about one's disability. Likewise, variations in one's culture and differences related to ethnicity can influence the interpretation of what constitutes good health (Freeman, 1998). From this framework, the interpreted concept of "good health" affects the response behavior when assessing health functioning using global markers of health.

Another possible explanation for differences in perception of functioning may be related to cultural variations on acceptable manifestations of illness. Although we did not find significant differences in rates of depression in our groups, reporting of physical ailments may be more acceptable for some cultures than mental illness. Earlier views of African Americans' attitude toward use of mental health services were accompanied with widespread shame, although this view is shifting (Dana, 1993). Sublimation of less desirable features associated with depression to physical disability may be more widely accepted by some minorities. Raskin and Mateer (2000) noted that physical exertion is often used by men as a means of coping with anger and anxiety. Associated feelings of awkwardness, balance problems, and reduced coordination from a mild TBI may adversely affect these customary methods of coping, possibly leading to feelings of lowered self-worth or esteem. Some may find it easier to admit to physical limitations than emotional dysfunction over which they may feel they have little control.

Incidence rates of MTBI is estimated at 262/100,000 for Hispanic Americans and at 278/100,000 for African Americans, with projected occurrence rates to be at 95,723 and 101,332, respectively, by the year 2010 (Cavallo & Saucedo, 1995; Cooper, Tabbador, Hauser, Shulman, Feiner, & Factor, 1993). Given these projected figures, health care professionals will be treating an increasingly large number of minority persons with an MTBI. Thus, studying the impact of culture or ethnicity on self-perceptions of health functioning becomes as important as studying the effects of age, sex, and socioeconomic status on outcome after MTBI. The interaction between culture and brain dysfunction may determine what experience is altered and how that experience is reported and expressed. The manifestation of a depressive disorder (and possibly other psychiatric disorders, including postconcussive disorder) may present differently in minority persons. Knowledge of cultural experiences and symptom presentation is warranted for treatment implications. Assessing mental and physical health functioning with African American and Hispanic American patients may require more in-depth interviewing to better understand any underlying or persisting symptomatology. Indicators of functional outcome and return to preinjury level of functioning, such as resumption of previous role activities, may not have the same level of significance in African American and Hispanic

American communities as it does in European American communities. Ability to perform household chores for African American and Hispanic patients may not be equated with the same level of significance as return to work, pain-free mobility, and mental health. Future studies may wish to consider the effect of these factors when assessing functional outcome.

References

Aitken, R. C. B. (1969). Measurement of feelings using the visual analogue scale. *Proceedings of the Royal Society of Medicine, 62,* 989–996.

Baker, S. P., O'Neill, B., Haddon, W., Jr., & Long, W. B. (1974). The injury severity score: A method for describing patients with multiple injuries and evaluating emergency care. *Journal of Trauma, 14,* 187–196.

Boyd, J. H., Weissman, M. M., Thompson, W. D., & Myers, J. K. (1982). Screening for depression in a community sample. *Archives of General Psychiatry, 39,* 1195–1200.

Brown, M., Gordon, W., & Haddad, L. (2000). Models for predicting subjective quality of life in individuals with traumatic brain injury. *Brain Injury, 14,* 5–19.

Bullinger, M., Azouvi, P., Brooks, N., Basso, A., Christensen, A., Gobiet, W., et al. (2002). Quality of life in patients with traumatic brain injury—Basic issues, assessment and recommendations. *Restorative Neurology and Neuroscience, 20,* 111–124.

Burnett, D., Silver, T., Kolakowsky-Hayner, S., & Cifu, D. (2000). Functional outcome for African Americans and Hispanics treated at a traumatic brain injury model systems centre. *Brain Injury, 14,* 713–718.

Cavallo, M. M., & Saucedo, C. (1995). Traumatic brain injury in families from culturally diverse populations. *J Head Traum Rehabil, 10,* 66–77.

Cooper, K. D., Tabbador, K., Hauser, W. A., Shulman, K., Feiner, C., & Factor, P. R. (1993). The epidemiology of head injury in the Bronx. *J Head Traum Rehabil, 2,* 70–78.

Corrigan, J. D., Smith-Knapp, K., & Granger, C. V. (1998). Outcomes in the first 5 years after traumatic brain injury. *Archives of Physical Medicine and Rehabilitation, 79,* 298–305.

Dacey, R., Dikmen, S., Temkin, N., McLean, A., Armsden, G., & Winn, H. (1991). Relative effects of brain and non-brain injuries on neuropsychological and psychosocial outcome. *Journal of Trauma, 31,* 217–222.

Dana, R. (1993). *Multicultural assessment perspectives for professional psychology.* Boston: Allyn & Bacon.

Deane, M., Pigott, T., & Dearing, P. (1996). The value of the Short Form 36 score in the outcome assessment of subarachnoid haemorrhage. *Br J Neurosurg, 10,* 187–191.

Dikmen, S., McLean, A., & Temkin, N. (1986). Neuropsychological and psychosocial consequences of minor head injury. *Journal of Neurology, Neurosurgery, and Psychiatry, 49,* 1227–1232.

Fann, J. R., Katon, W. J., Vomoto, J. M., & Esselman, P. C. (1995). Psychiatric disorders and functional disability in outpatients with traumatic brain injuries. *American Journal of Psychiatry, 152,* 1493–1499.

Fenton, G., McClelland, R., Montgomery, A., MacFlynn, G., & Rutherford, W. (1993). The postconcussional syndrome: Social antecedents and psychological sequelae. *Br J.Psychiatry, 162,* 493–497.

Findler, M., Cantor, J., Haddad, L., Gordon, W., & Ashman, T. (2001). The reliability and validity of the SF-36 health survey questionnaire for use with individuals with traumatic brain injury. *Brain Injury, 15,* 715–723.

First, M., Spitzer, R., Gibbon, M., & Williams, J. (1995). *User's guide for the structured clinical interview for DSM-IV Axis I Disorders–Research version (2nd ed.).* New York.

Freeman, H. (1998). The meaning of race in science—considerations for cancer research: Concerns of special populations in the National Cancer Program. *Cancer, 82,* 219–225.

Granger, C. V., Divan, N., & Fiedler, R. C. (1995). Functional assessment scales. A study of persons after traumatic brain injury. *American Journal of Physical Medicine and Rehabilitation, 74,* 107–113.

Jackson-Triche, M., Greer Sullivan, J., Wells, K., Rogers, W., Camp, P., & Mazel, R. (2000). Depression and health-related quality of life in ethnic minorities seeking care in general medical settings. *Journal of Affective Disorders, 58,* 89–97.

Levin, H., Mattis, S., Ruff, R., Eisenberg, H., Marshall, L., Tabaddor, K., et al. (1987). Neurobehavioral outcome following minor head injury: A three-center study. *Journal of Neurosurgery, 66,* 234–243.

Linn, M. W., Hunter, K. I., & Linn, B. S. (1980). Self-assessed health, impairment and disability in Anglo, Black and Cuban elderly. *Medical Care, 18,* 282–288.

Michaels, A. J., Michaels, C. E., Moon, C. H., Smith, J. S., Zimmerman, M. A., Taheri, P. A., et al. (1999). Posttraumatic stress disorder after injury: Impact on general health outcome and early risk assessment. *Journal of Trauma, 47,* 460–466.

Michaels, A. J., Michaels, C. E., Smith, J. S., Moon, C. H., Peterson, C., & Long, W. B. (2000). Outcome from injury: General health, work status, and satisfaction 12 months after trauma. *J Trauma, 48,* 841–850.

Paniak, C., Phillips, K., Toller-Lobe, G., Durand, A., & Nagy, J. (1999). Sensitivity of three recent questionnaires to mild traumatic brain injury-related effects. *Journal of Head Trauma Rehabilitation, 14,* 211–219.

Ponsford, J., Willmott, C., Rothwell, A., Cameron, P., Kelly, A. M., Nelms, R., et al. (2000). Factors influencing outcome following mild traumatic brain injury in adults. *Journal of International Neuropsychology Society, 6,* 568–579.

Prigatano, G. (1999). *Principles of neuropsychological rehabilitation.* New York: Oxford University Press.

Radloff, L. S. (1977). The CES-D Scale: A self-report depression scale for research in the general population. *Applied Psychological Measurement, 1,* 385–401.

Raskin, S., & Mateer, C. (2000). Issues of gender, socioeconomic status, and culture. In S. Raskin & C. Mateer (Eds.), *Neuropsychological management of mild traumatic brain injury* (pp. 269–278). New York: Oxford University Press.

Ren, X. S., & Amick, B. C. (1996). Racial and ethnic disparities in self-assessed health status: Evidence from the National Survey of Families and Households. *Ethnic Health, 1,* 293–303.

Rimel, R., Giordani, B., Barth, J., & Jane, J. (1982). Moderate head injury: Completing the clinical spectrum of brain trauma. *Neurosurgery, 11,* 344–351.

Rosenthal, M., Dijkers, M., Harrison-Felix, C., Nabors, N., Witol, A., Young, M. E., et al. (1996). Impact of minority status on functional outcome and community integration following traumatic brain injury. *Journal of Head Trauma Rehabilitation, 11,* 40–57.

Sarason, I. G., Sarason, B. R., Shearin, E. N., et al. (1987). A brief measure of social support: Practical and theoretical implications. *Journal of Social and Personal Relations, 4,* 497–510.

Shetterly, S., Baxter, J., Mason, L., & Hamman, R. (1996). Self-rated health among Hispanic vs non-Hispanic white adults: The San Luis Valley Health and Aging Study. *American Journal of Public Health, 86,* 1798–1801.

Simpson, G., Mohr, G., & Redman, A. (2000). Cultural variations in the understanding of traumatic brain injury and brain injury rehabilitation. *Brain Injury., 14,* 125–140.

Teasdale, G., & Jennett, B. (1974). Assessment of coma and impaired consciousness. A practical scale. *Lancet, 2,* 81–84.

Ware, J. E., Jr., & Sherbourne, C. D. (1992). The MOS 36-item Short-Form Health Survey (SF-36): I. Conceptual framework and item selection. *Medical Care, 30,* 473–483.

Willer, B., Rosenthal, M., Kreutzer, J. S., Gordon, W. A., & Rempel, R. (1993). Assessment of community integration following rehabilitation for traumatic brain injury. *Journal of Head Trauma Rehabilitation, 8,* 75–87.

T - #0161 - 160425 - C0 - 280/208/4 - PB - 9780805895575 - Gloss Lamination

APPLIED NEUROPSYCHOLOGY

Table of Contents
VOLUME 11 • NUMBER 1 • 2004

Special Issue: Cultural Diversity
Ruben J. Echemendia, Guest Editor

INTRODUCTION

Cultural Diversity and Neuropsychology: An Uneasy Relationship in a Time of Change.....................1
  Ruben J. Echemendia

ARTICLES

Neuropsychological Test Use With Hispanic/Latino Populations in the United States:
Part II of a National Survey...4
  Ruben J. Echemendia and Josette G. Harris

Racial and Ethnic Diversity Among Trainees and Professionals in Psychology and Neuropsychology:
Needs, Trends, and Challenges..13
  Felicia Hill-Briggs, Jovier D. Evans, and Marc A. Norman

Neuropsychological Assessment of Asian Americans: Demographic Factors, Cultural Diversity,
and Practical Guidelines...23
  Tony M. Wong and Daryl E. Fujii

Acculturation, Reading Level, and Neuropsychological Test Performance Among African American Elders....37
  Jennifer J. Manly, Desiree A. Byrd, Pegah Touradji, and Yaakov Stern

Differences in Neuropsychological Performance Associated With Ethnicity in Children With HIV-1 Infection:
Preliminary Findings...47
  Antolin M. Llorente, Marie Turcich, and Kelly A. Lawrence

Perception of Health and Quality of Life in Minorities After Mild-to-Moderate Traumatic Brain Injury........54
  Sharon A. Brown, Stephen R. McCauley, Harvey S. Levin, Charles Contant, and Corwin Boake

ISBN 978-0-8058-9557-5
90000

9 780805 895575

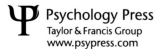

Psychology Press
Taylor & Francis Group
www.psypress.com

Volume 9, Number 2

2000

Journal of

CONSUMER PSYCHOLOGY

The Official Journal of
The Society for Consumer Psychology

Special Issue:

Cultural Psychology

Guest Editors:

Durairaj Maheswaran
Sharon Shavitt

EDITORS

Paul M. Herr
University of Colorado, Boulder

Frank R. Kardes
University of Cincinnati

ASSOCIATE EDITOR

Curtis P. Haugtvedt
Ohio State University

EDITOR ELECT

Dawn Iacobucci
Northwestern University